Clinics in Human Lactation

Breastfeeding after Breast and Nipple Procedures:

A Guide for Healthcare Professionals

Diana West, BA, IBCLC and Elliot M. Hirsch, MD

Clinics in Human Lactation

Breastfeeding after Breast and Nipple Procedures: A Guide for Healthcare Professionals

Diana West, BA, IBCLC and Elliot M. Hirsch, MD

Praeclarus Press, LLC
2504 Sweetgum Lane
Amarillo, Texas 79124 USA
806-367-9950
www.PraeclarusPress.com

DISCLAIMER
The information contained in this publication is advisory only and is not intended to replace sound clinical judgment or individualized patient care. The author disclaims all warranties, whether expressed or implied, including any warranty as the quality, accuracy, safety, or suitability of this information for any particular purpose.

ISBN: 978-1-939807-82-3

TABLE OF CONTENTS

Breastfeeding after Breast and Nipple Procedures: A Guide for Healthcare Professionals

---

PURPOSE

The purpose of this guide is to provide the healthcare professional with an understanding of breast and nipple surgeries and their effects upon lactation and the breastfeeding relationship. This guide has delineated discussion of breastfeeding after breast and nipple surgeries according to three broad categories: diagnostic, ablative, and therapeutic breast procedures; cosmetic breast surgeries; and nipple surgeries. The reasons, motivations, issues, concerns, stresses, and physical and psychological results share some commonalities, but they are largely unique to the type of surgery performed. For this reason, each type of surgery and its effect upon lactation will be discussed independently. Methods to assess milk production and an overview of feeding options to maximize milk production when supplementation is necessary are presented. The role of the healthcare professional in assisting mothers to breastfeed after breast and nipple surgeries is discussed and resources are included. A glossary is provided for definition of unfamiliar anatomical or surgical terms.

INTRODUCTION

The lactation functionality that remains after breast and nipple surgeries depends primarily upon the character of the incisions and dissections, the degree of destruction of parenchyma, and the extent of damage to nerves critical to lactation. It is also affected by the functionality of the parenchyma prior to surgery, the post-operative course, the time interval between the surgery and the lactation event, other lactation experiences between the surgery and the lactation event, breastfeeding management, as well as the mother's attitude toward breastfeeding. In short, any surgery to the breast or nipple can alter lactation functionality.

From the clinical perspective, working with patients who are breastfeeding with reduced functionality can seem to be a risk to the infant's adequate intake. When a treatment plan is implemented according to the principles described in this guide, however, this risk can be minimized. The most important of these principles is that the parents remain vigilant, constantly monitoring the physiological health of their babies in collaboration with a healthcare provider in order to provide early warning of impending infant deterioration.

A satisfying breastfeeding relationship is not precluded by insufficient milk production. When measures are taken to protect the milk supply that exists, minimize supplementation, and increase milk production when possible, a mother with compromised milk production can have a satisfying breastfeeding relationship with her baby.

PREDICTING LACTATION CAPABILITY AFTER BREAST AND NIPPLE PROCEDURES

The aspect of breast and nipple procedures that is most likely to affect lactation is the surgical treatment of the parenchyma and nipple-areola complex. The location, orientation, and length of the incision and dissection may directly affect lactation capability by damaging the parenchyma and innervation to the nipple/areolar complex. An incision near or on the areola, particularly in the lower, outer quadrant of the areola, is more likely to damage the fourth intercostal nerve, which is critical to lactation (Neifert, 1992). A horizontal incision across the breast may be more likely to injure lactation tissue than a vertical incision that is parallel to the ducts. An incision in the outer and lower portions of the breast may be more damaging to lactation capability because this is where the nerves critical to milk ejection are located (Schlenz et al., 2000), and milk ejection is essential to milk removal (Ramsay et al., 2004).

When women consult a surgeon prior to breast surgery, they are often advised that the surgery will affect their lactation capability to some degree. Depending on the surgery, doctors commonly describe the potential capability by stating that there is either no possibility that the woman will be able to lactate after the surgery, a "50/50" chance, or that it will not affect her lactation capability at all (Nommsen-Rivers, 2003). A surgeon's projections of lactation capability, however, are often based on the assumption that any lactation is *full* lactation and may fail to quantify the volume of the mother's milk production.

The "50/50" chance frequently quoted usually refers to the surgeon's estimate of a 50 percent probability that she will be able to lactate at all. A woman may be incorrectly informed that if she has any milk, she will be able to exclusively breastfeed, or that if she has no milk, she will not be able to breastfeed at all. The critical information for a future mother, however, is not whether she will be able to lactate at all, but rather how much she will be able to lactate, as almost all mothers who have had breast and nipple surgeries are able to produce some amount of milk (barring mastectomy or radiation) (Harris et al., 1992). Because their probable lactation capability was described in absolute terms, some mothers mistakenly think that if they are able to express any colostrum or milk, then they will produce a full milk supply. Conversely, if they cannot express colostrum during pregnancy or they do not see any milk in the first few days postpartum, they may think they are completely unable to lactate. Many mothers do not understand that the process of lactation, especially after breast and nipple surgeries, is more complex than these basic assumptions.

EFFECTS OF TISSUE REGENERATION UPON LACTATION CAPABILITY

Recanalization is an important physiological phenomenon for women who have had breast surgery. It is the process wherein breast tissue is regrown, reconnecting previously severed ducts or connecting new ductal pathways.

Any duration of lactation seems to prompt the mammary system to reestablish new ducts. Lactation tissue is also formed in response to hormones that occur during menstruation. Therefore, the longer the mother has lactated and the more menstrual cycles she has experienced after surgery, the greater the extent of recanalization. A mother whose previous lactation efforts resulted in an incomplete supply may find that subsequent attempts result in a much greater yield. In some mothers, recanalization has resulted in a complete milk supply for subsequent children.

Reinnervation is the process whereby damaged nerves regenerate. The fourth intercostal nerve is the nerve that most consistently innervates the nipple/areolar complex and thus is critical to the process of lactation because stimulation of this nerve triggers the release of oxytocin, which causes milk ejection. Regeneration of this critical neural pathway becomes a key component in increased lactation

3

capability. The process of reinnervation is not influenced by previous lactation events, but depends primarily on the extent of nerve damage and the location of the injury. Nerves that are completely transected will undergo Wallerian degeneration and regrow at a predictable rate of one inch per month after an initial month of degeneration and recovery, typically taking at least six months to one year to fully regenerate, depending on the distance of the injury from the neural cell body (Shaw et al., 1997). If women regain response to touch and temperature, this indicates the fourth intercostal nerve is functioning and will conduct the appropriate sensations to the pituitary gland for production of prolactin and oxytocin. Of course, the ability of the mammary system to fulfill the demand is dependent upon the state of the glands and ducts. Nonetheless, the longer the length of time since the surgery, the greater the chances that the nerves critical to lactation have regenerated.

EFFECTS OF DIAGNOSTIC, ABLATIVE, AND THERAPEUTIC PROCEDURES UPON LACTATION FUNCTIONALITY

A woman who has been identified as having fibrocystic disease, a cyst (solid or fluid-filled), or a lump may be referred to a breast surgeon for diagnosis and treatment. Diagnosis and treatment may require imaging techniques, ductogram, aspiration, biopsy, or removal of the suspected tissue. Treatment for cardiac and pulmonary dysfunction may also require surgery through the mammary tissue. The effect of the diagnostic or therapeutic procedure upon lactation capability is dependent upon the type of procedure and the state of lactation.

Imaging Techniques

Imaging techniques used for diagnosis of breast pathology include ultrasound, mammogram, magnetic resonance imaging (MRI), positron emission tomography (PET) scan, 2-Methoxy Isobutyl Isonitrile (MIBI) scan, electrical impedance tomography (EIT) scan, computed tomography (CT) scan (also known as computer axial tomography (CAT) scan), thermography, or diaphanography. Imaging techniques are non-invasive and do not affect lactation capability.

Ductogram

In performing a ductogram, a fine plastic catheter is inserted into a lactation duct through the nipple. A radioactive dye is injected through the catheter into the duct and an x-ray is taken to produce an image. An endoscopy also may be performed. In this procedure, a minute camera is inserted into the ducts in order to visualize the internal ductal walls (Escobar et al., 2004). As no incisions or excisions are made during this procedure, there is generally no impact upon lactation capability.

Needle Aspiration

Needle aspiration is a diagnostic procedure used to remove the cellular contents of fluid-filled cysts and galactoceles. In fine needle aspiration, a small needle is injected directly into several locations above the location of the cyst and the contents of the cyst are drawn into the needle. Bruising and minor bleeding into the cyst are common after aspiration. As the parenchymal trauma is minimal, there is generally no impact upon lactation capability.

Biopsy

Biopsy to remove tissue for diagnostic analysis carries the inherent risk of severing lactation ducts or nerves. It may be performed with a fine or large needle, or it may be incisional or excisional, depending on the size of the suspected mass and other factors. Diagnostic biopsy may include the affected alveolus and ductules. If the analyzed tissue is malignant, a partial or full mastectomy may be performed.

Core (needle or Tru-Cut) biopsy is a procedure that uses a larger needle to remove a core of tissue from the center of a cyst. There are several methods of obtaining a core biopsy. Frequently, a small incision is made above the cyst and the needle is passed through the incision. Several tissue samples are withdrawn for analysis.

Stereotactic biopsy is a procedure that isolates the precise location of a suspected mass using computers and radiographic images taken from multiple angles. One type of this procedure employs an advanced breast biopsy instrument (ABBI), which uses a very large needle, resulting in a large incision that often requires suturing. A mammotome (MIBB) is another instrument that removes tissue by suction. This process removes greater amounts of tissue than standard needle biopsy. Core biopsies can also be taken with a hand-held device, guided by ultrasound.

When a mass has been identified on mammography and cannot be identified on physical exam, a wire localization biopsy procedure may be performed by inserting a needle into the breast through which a thin wire is attached. The wire, guided radiographically, is positioned at the site of the suspected mass, and the surgeon uses the wire to locate and remove the mass.

The impact upon lactation from biopsy depends upon the surgical approach of the biopsy and the amount of nerve and parenchyma disruption. Scarring or the complication of an infection or hematoma subsequent to a biopsy may have an effect upon lactation, depending on the extent. Many surgeons attempt to preserve the aesthetic integrity of the breast by placing incisions in less visible areas, such as around the areola or under the inframammary fold. When the incision is placed a distance from the mass, the surgeon must dissect the breast parenchyma more extensively to reach the mass, which increases the risk of severed ducts and lactation disruption. An incision on or around the perimeter of the areola may result in reduced innervation to the nipple/areolar complex, thus reducing the neurohormonal lactation response. When the suspected mass resides under the areola or in the nipple, such as in Paget's disease, incisions that damage the nipple/areolar complex are unavoidable. Orienting them toward the upper and inner quadrants will theoretically reduce the likelihood of nerve impairment (Pezzi et al., 2004).

Mastectomy

In some circumstances, mastectomy may be necessary. When the surgery is unilateral and occurs during active lactation, and if the mother desires to do

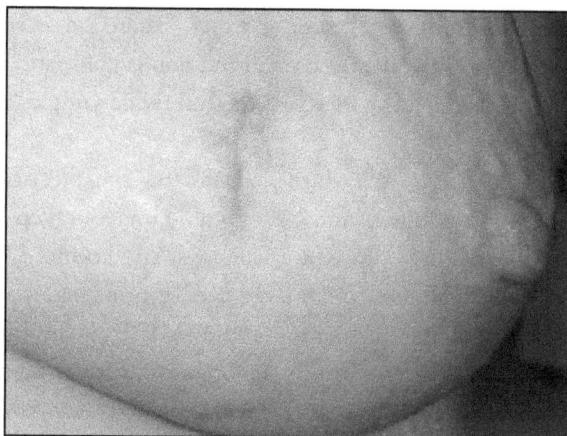

Figure 1. Biopsy scar - four months post-op (Photo courtesy of Diana West)

so, she can continue to breastfeed on the contralateral breast (Mohrbacher, 2004). By employing protocols to increase milk production, it is possible that full milk production can be achieved on that side. If full milk production does not develop, supplementation can be given in a manner that is supportive of breastfeeding (see below) so that the breastfeeding relationship is preserved.

Sternotomy

Surgery through the breast to treat cardiac or pulmonary dysfunction necessarily carries the risk of lactation impairment. In order to preserve lactation function and minimize scarring, it is common for the incision to be placed in the inframammary fold (transverse submammary incision) (Nakamura et al., 1997; Bedard et al., 1986; Brutel de la Riviere et al., 1981). A study in 1993 by Deutinger and Deutinger examined the effects of breastfeeding after cardiac surgery when the incision is through the inframammary fold, and found that breastfeeding did not complicate healing. An earlier study in 1992 by Deutinger and Dominag reported excellent lactation outcomes when the incision for sternotomy is made in the inframammary fold (Deutinger & Dominag, 1992). This is likely to be a consistent finding, although consideration must be given to the extent of the surgery and post-operative healing. Even when the incision is in the inframammary fold, ductal pathways can be severed. Post-operative infection or other complications, such as seroma or hematoma, can also impede lactation function.

Necessity for Interruption of Breastfeeding

It is common for mothers to be instructed to suspend breastfeeding for days, weeks, or months prior to diagnostic imaging, aspiration, or biopsy. Diagnostic imaging techniques are more difficult to interpret during lactation, due to the increased density of breast tissue, but it is not impossible to do so. In addition, although surgeons may be reluctant to perform breast biopsies in women who are lactationally active, the current literature does not support the view that breastfeeding is an absolute contraindication to breast biopsy, nor does it support the theory that active lactation leads to delayed wound healing (Buescher, 2001). There is a risk of duct/nerve damage during breast biopsy, which may lead to difficulties with lactation. Also, there is a definite risk of a galactocele, which will probably drain through the skin and may lead to increased risk of infection, although this point is controversial.

From the surgical perspective, visualization of the surgical field in a lactationally active breast will be more obscured, which may make an accurate biopsy difficult to obtain. The preferable approach to biopsy in this situation is a stereotactic biopsy or fine needle aspiration whenever possible. However, in the event that an open biopsy is absolutely necessary, the final decision as to whether or not to wean prior to biopsy is individualized, and should be made after a discussion with the doctor, during which the risks and benefits are explained. If the surgeon is not comfortable doing the procedure without weaning and the mother insists on continuing to breastfeed, she should go to another surgeon.

In addition, it is important to consider that abrupt weaning can be psychologically traumatic for both the mother and her nursling, without regard to the child's age. It also introduces the possibility of plugged ducts and infectious mastitis from sudden milk stasis. No matter how abruptly milk removal is ceased, milk can continue to be produced for many months. For this reason, there is almost certain to be residual milk in the ducts when surgery is performed on a recently lactating woman. A breast that has been thoroughly drained by nursing or pumping immediately prior to the diagnostic or ablative surgery will minimize milk seepage during the procedure.

Anesthesia and Analgesia

When injected into the skin for superficial procedures, local anesthetic medications do not transfer into milk in clinically relevant levels. There is no need for a mother to interrupt breastfeeding when local anesthetic medications have been used (Hale, 1999; Hale, 2008).

It is safe for a mother to nurse her baby or pump her milk as soon as she awakens fully from general anesthesia, as anesthetic medications have brief plasma half-lives and are rapidly metabolized. When the mother is no longer drowsy, the anesthetic medications are no longer active in her milk (Spigset, 1994; Hale, 1999; Hale, 2008).

Women should consult their anesthesiologist to discuss appropriate post-operative pain medication, referring to the bi-annually revised *Medications and Mothers' Milk* by Dr. Thomas Hale (Hale Publishing) or other similar resources to determine the compatibility of such drugs with breastfeeding.

Effects of Diagnostic Procedures upon Milk Safety

Ultrasound procedures do not affect the quality or safety of the milk and are wholly compatible with breastfeeding.

Radiation and radioactive agents are common tools used in diagnostic procedures. The compatibility of the radioactive procedure with breastfeeding depends upon the type of radiation used. The effects of an x-ray can be likened to using a flash while taking a photograph; after the x-ray is taken, the radiation is no longer present in the same way that the light from a camera is no longer present after the flash has discharged. Thus, x-rays, mammograms, MRI, and CT scans are all safe during lactation. It is not uncommon for mothers to be advised to "pump and dump" their milk for an arbitrary period of time subsequent to mammographic testing. This is not necessary. While x-ray radiation does have the ability to mutate DNA in live cells, it does not collect in the milk and is therefore compatible with uninterrupted breastfeeding.

The radiopaque and radiocontrast agents typically used in the ductogram, CT, MRI, MIBI scan, or PET scan diagnostic tests are extremely inert and are virtually unabsorbed after oral administration (Hale, 2008). Several studies have failed to find any negative effects among babies who have ingested milk subsequent to radioactive agent imaging procedures (Kubik-Hutch, 2000; Nielsen et al., 1987). Consequently, it is not necessary to interrupt breastfeeding when radiopaque and radiocontrast agents are used in imaging procedures (Kubik-Hutch et al., 2000; Rofsky et al., 1993; Nielsen et al., 1987; FitzJohn et al., 1982).

Radioactive agents contain particulate radiation, which consists of atoms with unstable nuclei that release radiation when they deteriorate. Certain types of these agents are uptaken by specific tissues and can thus detect metabolic and structural features. Ingestion or injection of a radioactive agent results in radiation residing in the body until the radiation completely degrades or is excreted. Consumption or injection of particulate radiation during lactation will result in transference of radioactive substances into the milk during milk synthesis. The radioactive toxicity and compatibility with breastfeeding depends upon the substance used.

The use of radioactive isotopes during diagnostic testing or therapy is contraindicated during breastfeeding, as such compounds accumulate in milk and are therefore hazardous to the infant. It is not necessary for mothers to wean with the intention of complete cessation of breastfeeding in order to undergo a procedure employing radioactive isotopes. She need only interrupt breastfeeding temporarily, feeding her infant previously pumped milk or formula until her milk is demonstrated by testing to be no longer radioactive (most hospital radiology departments are able to perform the tests). Frequent pumping during this time will protect her milk supply and accelerate removal of radiation from her body (Mohrbacher, 2004).

Radiation Therapy

Therapy with pure energy radiation is injurious to all breast and chest wall tissue, including the parenchyma. This effect is usually permanent (Neifert, 1992; David, 1985; Higgins & Haffty, 1994) and consequently an irradiated breast is likely to produce a substantially reduced milk supply, even to the point of no milk at all. However, lactation will be unaffected on the breast that did not receive radiation. If radiation therapy is administered during active lactation, the mother can continue to breastfeed on the contralateral breast (Mohrbacher, 2004). By employing protocols to increase milk production, it is possible that a full milk supply can be achieved on that side. If full milk production does not develop, supplementation can be given in a manner that is supportive of breastfeeding (see below), so that the breastfeeding relationship is preserved.

CHEMOTHERAPY

Breastfeeding during chemotherapy is almost always contraindicated, as the medications used to eradicate cancer are highly toxic and transfer into milk (Hale, 2008; Helewa et al., 2002). Breastfeeding may continue in some cases after the use of various chemotherapeutic medications, but not all of them. Most chemotherapeutic agents are rapidly cleared from the body, and in these instances, mothers can resume breastfeeding safely. Physicians should consult a resource that addresses drugs and breastfeeding, such as the chemotherapy appendix in *Medications and Mothers' Milk*, with regard to the initiation and duration of weaning, as these factors vary among different chemotherapeutic agents.

Breastfeeding and Cancer

Many myths have been perpetuated about breastfeeding when a mother has cancer or after her cancer has been removed. For instance, mothers have been warned that cancer can be transmitted to their babies by suckling a cancerous breast. This has never been documented in humans and is highly unlikely. Another myth is that a baby will refuse to suckle a cancerous breast. This is not necessary true, although babies have been known to occasionally refuse a breast when the milk changes taste or the milk supply decreases as a result of a malignant mass (Tralins, 1995). There is no evidence that breastfeeding increases the risk of breast cancer recurrence or that it carries any health risk to the child (Helewa et al., 2002).

A mother with cancer may be told that weaning is necessary in order to "conserve her strength." However, breastfeeding is considerably more convenient and less time-consuming than bottle-feeding. More importantly, it provides an emotional connection and intimacy that is nurturing to both mother and baby when they need it most.

EFFECTS OF COSMETIC BREAST SURGERIES UPON LACTATION FUNCTIONALITY

Augmentation Mammaplasty

The psychological motivations to undergo this surgery are as compelling as the physical. A 2003 study by Didie and Sarwer examined the factors that motivate women to seek cosmetic breast augmentation surgery, and found that breast augmentation patients were more motivated by their feelings about their breasts than by influences from external sources, such as romantic partners or sociocultural representations of beauty (Didie & Sarwer, 2003). Other studies have shown that certain augmentation mammaplasty techniques can improve body image (Banbury et al., 2004). This clearly refutes the common stereotype of the narcissistic woman with breast implants. In *Surgery of the Breast: Principles and Art* (Spear, 2006), it is noted:

Descriptions of women seeking augmentation mammaplasty are very consistent, with a common thread being their doubts about their femininity, which motivate them to request the surgery. It is further postulated that preoccupation with breast size in women seeking augmentation mammaplasty does not arise suddenly, but usually either dates to adolescence or develops after childbirth. Among women seeking augmentation mammaplasty, there is a higher incidence of divorce, unhappy marriages, emotional discomfort, diminished feelings of femininity, and elevated levels of depression than in the general population. Most women seeking augmentation mammaplasty do so while in their thirties and are likely to report concerns about their appearance and preoccupation with inadequate breast size. Most women are not seeking to outdo other women in breast size; rather they want to catch up.

In considering lactation capability, the original state of the breasts prior to augmentation is a critical determiner of inherent lactation potential, even before the impact of surgery. Although small breast size alone is not a marker for lactation insufficiency, certain breast types are known to be markers for hypoplasia (Neifert et al., 1985). These types include tubular-shaped breasts, widely spaced breasts, undeveloped breasts, such as Poland's Syndrome, and asymmetrical breasts. When so little parenchyma exists, lactation capability can be significantly diminished. Most women report that they are not advised that they may have an inherent hypoplasia or that augmentation mammaplasty can reduce lactation capability (Spear, 2005).

As with all breast surgeries, the surgical approach dictates the impact upon lactation (Neifert, 1992). The nipple-areolar complex is most reliably innervated by branches of the fourth intercostal nerve. The lateral branch of this

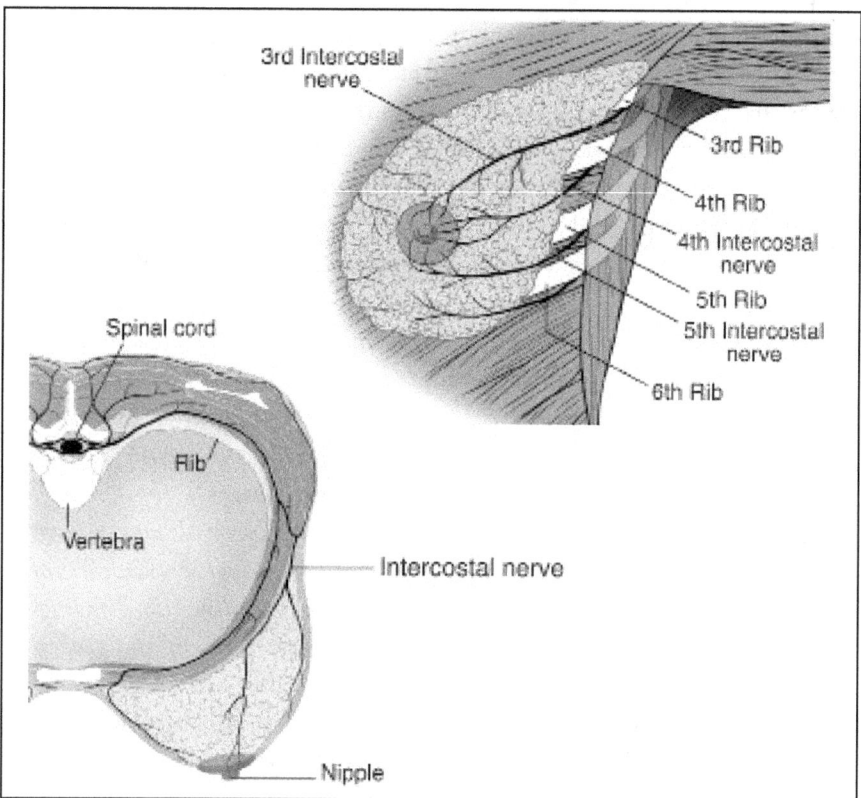

Figure 2. Innervation of the breast. (Illustration copyright © Taina Litwak, CMI. Used with permission.)

nerve tends to enter the nipple from the posterior direction, while the anterior cutaneous branch typically reaches the areola between the 8:00 and 11:00 positions on the left and 1:00 to 4:00 positions on the right (Schlenz, 2000). Thus, surgical approaches in these areas have a higher chance of damaging these nerves and interfering with lactation. With regard to breast augmentation, periareolar incisions have a higher likelihood of damaging the nerves that innervate the nipple-areolar complex, and thus may be more likely to decrease the chances of successful lactation (Brody, 1996). This was examined in a study by Hurst in 1996, which found that not only was augmentation mammaplasty in general associated with decreased lactation outcome, but specifically women with a periareolar incision had a statistically significant decrease in sufficient lactation. However, several confounding variables were not addressed in this study, including implant size, pocket position, and surgical dissection after the initial incision. If the dissection to the pectoralis fascia is performed through a direct anterior to posterior approach, there will be more duct damage and thus a higher risk to lactation. It is probable that these factors affected the results of the Hurst study, especially considering recent studies that have found no statistically significant difference in nipple sensitivity between periareolar incisions and inframammary fold incisions (Modfid et al., 2006). Interestingly, the Modfid study found a statistically significant association between increased implant size and decreased nipple sensation, which may have been due to nerve traction injury caused by the larger implants. As the link between lactation outcomes and breast augmentation approach has not been definitively examined, when considering breast augmentation in women who may become pregnant and breastfeed, it may be preferable to avoid a periareolar incision. When the patient has been informed of the potential risks of this incision and still chooses it for her surgery, surgeons should consider tunneling subcutaneously through the lower pole of the breast, rather than dissecting directly in the anterior-posterior direction, to reach the pectoralis muscle in order to reduce trauma to the breast parenchyma and nerves. Finally, women who are undergoing breast augmentation should be advised that increased implant size may decrease nipple sensitivity and potentially impact lactation.

Placement of the implant can also theoretically affect lactation functionality. Although no studies to date have directly examined the effect implant placement has on lactation outcome, authors have suggested that subglandular implant positioning under the parenchyma and above the pectoralis muscle is more likely to put pressure on the parenchyma and thereby compromise milk production than a submuscular implant positioning (Michalopoulos, 2007; Hurst, 1996). However, the vast majority of breast augmentations today are performed in the submuscular plane or through a biplanar approach (a combination of submuscular and subglandular), and as such, this potential problem is less of an issue.

It is important to note that augmentation mammaplasty is frequently revised because of breast ptosis, desired size change, implant deflation (with saline implants), scar revision, and capsular contracture. Complications, such as hematoma, seroma, and infection, may also necessitate reoperation. The average duration to revision is seven years (Spears et al., 2003). Revision surgeries may damage nerves and breast parenchyma, and consequently may negatively impact lactation capability (Michalopoulos, 2007, Henriksen, 2003). Revisions from capsular contracture, in particular, can damage nerves and breast parenchyma, and thus can decrease milk production (Michalopoulos, 2007, Strom et al., 1997).

Another interesting but rare complication following breast augmentation is post-surgical galactorrhea, which was documented by Caputy and Flowers in a 1994 study. The galactorrhea spontaneously developed an average of 6.6 days post-operatively and was self-limited with an average duration of 5.2 days. The only statistically significant factor associated with the galactorrhea was gravidity of the patient. The relationship between the galactorrhea and mature lactation following pregnancy was not investigated (Caputy & Flowers, 1994).

Effects of Silicone Transfer into Milk

Well-publicized reports in previous decades of concerns about the transfer of silicone into human milk have raised public awareness of this issue. However, recent studies have shown that, "...lactating women with silicone implants are similar to control women with respect to levels of silicon in their breast milk and blood. Silicon levels are ten times higher in cow's milk, and even higher in infant formulas" (Semple et al., 1998). In a 1994 study by Berlin, it was noted, "...silicone is widely present in the environment and avoiding ingestion is difficult. Silicone drops have been used for years in both the US and Europe for colic." This study concluded that there should be no absolute contraindication to breastfeeding by women with silicone breast implants (Berlin, 1994). It is also reassuring to note that silicone is considered inert and unlikely to be absorbed by the baby's digestive tract (Hale, 2008).

Common Augmentation Mammaplasty Techniques

The purpose of these different approaches is to minimize visible scarring. The actual size of the incision is highly variable and depends on the surgeon's preference. Generally, the size of the incision is made as small as possible, but still allows good pocket visualization and accurate implant placement. The discussion of the surgical approaches that follows in this monograph are highly simplified and are described based on their relevance to lactation.

Inframammary Fold Augmentation Mammaplasty

The inframammary fold approach is a common breast augmentation approach and works well for both subglandular and subpectoral implant placement. Dissection to the pectoralis major from this incision largely avoids the parenchyma and preserves nipple/areolar innervation.

This approach begins with an incision at the site of what is anticipated to be the new inframammary fold. Next, the surgeon dissects through the subcutaneous fat and parenchyma to the pectoralis major. A pocket is developed for the implant, which is then inserted and filled. By filling the implant after placing it in the pocket, the surgeon can use a smaller incision. If gel implants are used, the incision may be slightly longer as they are pre-filled. Once placement and filling of the implant is complete, the incision is closed.

Transaxillary Approach

The transaxillary approach involves the use of an endoscope in order to facilitate accurate implant placement. The incision is made in the first axillary crease, posterior to the anterior axillary line. The subcutaneous tissue is dissected, and the pectoralis muscle is approached laterally. Commonly, this muscle is incised laterally, and the endoscope is inserted from this direction. Next, under endoscopic visualization, a pocket is created to receive the implant. The implant is then inserted, filled, and the incisions are closed.

Transumbilical Endoscopic Augmentation (TUBA Mammaplasty

The transumbilical technique, commonly called Transumbilical Breast Augmentation (TUBA), is performed by first making an incision in the umbilicus, and then using an endoscope to tunnel through the subcutaneous tissue of the abdominal wall into the breast. Next, the implant pocket is created, and finally the implant is tunneled into place in the breast. In this technique, no incisions are made percutaneously into the breast, although the breast parenchyma is dissected to create the implant pocket. Even with the use of an endoscope, it is difficult to create the pocket for the implant, and if complications, such as hematoma, develop, it is frequently necessary to open the breast pocket through an inframammary or periareolar incision (Kryger & Sisco, 2007). This technique is the least frequently utilized of the breast augmentation approaches.

Periareolar Approach

In the periareolar approach, an incision is made in a semi-circle around the lower part of the areola. The dissection either proceeds directly through the breast parenchyma to the pectoralis major, or is carried out by tunneling through the subcutaneous tissues of the lower pole of the breast down to the pectoralis major. A pocket is then created in the desired plane, after which the implant is inserted and filled, and the incision is closed.

Reduction Mammaplasty

Reduction mammaplasty is surgery to reduce the size and volume of the breast. There are many reasons why women with hypertrophic breasts undergo reduction mammaplasty, and include both physical and psychological factors. Women with mammary hypertrophy may suffer from back or shoulder pain, neuromuscular dysfunction, including headaches and nerve damage, and may also suffer from postural difficulties. In addition, due to the large size of their breasts, these women are often limited in their physical activities. The breasts rubbing against each other may cause intertriginous lesions on the medial sides of the breasts, and it is not uncommon for women with hypertrophic breasts to have frequent yeast infections in the inframammary fold, as well as premature, exaggerated ptosis.

As with augmentation surgery, psychological factors likely play a role in influencing women to undergo reduction mammaplasty, although women may be reluctant to discuss this candidly. These women may feel tremendous pressure to look normal and "fit in." In a society that equates large breasts with promiscuity, a young woman with hypertrophic breasts may attract unwanted attention that may make her feel very uncomfortable. Women who undergo breast reduction at a young age may not be trying to achieve aesthetic perfection as much as they are trying to feel more normal, and may not be concerned about breast function at the time of their surgeries (Aillet et al., 2002). Because their physical appearance differs so greatly from their peers, young women with hypertropic breasts may have a poor self-image and perceive themselves as having a physical abnormality. Reduction mammaplasty can transform their bodies into the range of normal and can significantly redeem their self-esteem. Among other surgical procedures on the breast, the American Society of Plastic Surgeons (ASPS) cites breast reduction as having one of the highest degrees of satisfaction (Collins et al., 2002).

There are many different surgical approaches to reduction mammaplasty. In order to understand the basis of these procedures, it is important to consider the blood supply to the nipple-areola complex. The nipple-areola complex is supplied by perforating arteries from the external and internal mammary arteries, as well as by perforating branches from the anterolateral and anteromedial intercostal arteries (Nahai, 2008). These blood vessels anastamose in a subdermal plexus circumferentially around the areola. Thus, the goal of breast reduction surgery is to remove breast tissue while keeping intact a predetermined radius of tissue, known as the pedicle, which will provide the blood supply to the nipple-areola complex. There are a variety of different pedicles that can be used, and these can be accessed through several different approaches. Consequently, scars differ widely according to the technique used, but in general can include a scar around the areola, vertical scars from the areolar to the inframammary fold of varying sizes, horizontal scars along the inframammary fold of varying sizes, or combinations of the above.

Regardless of the surgical approach used, some amount of breast tissue will be removed. Depending on the amount of tissue, location of removal, and extent of damage to the remaining breast structures, lactation may be

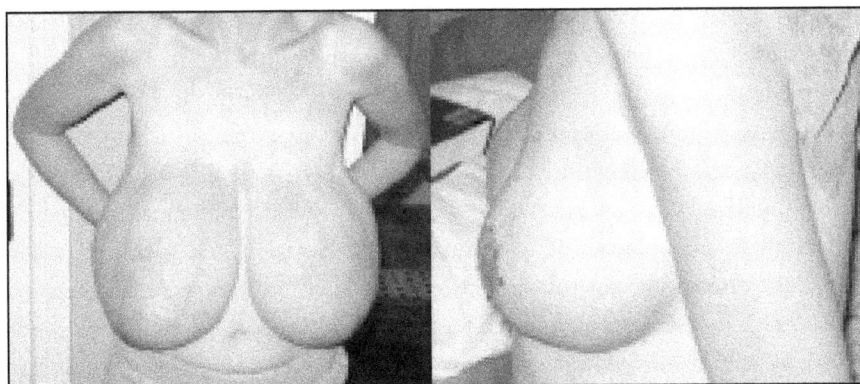

Figure 3. Gigantomastia - Patient grew to bra size 44L during pregnancy, shown here (left) after delivery at size 36G; after reduction surgery (right), she was bra size 34B. (Photo courtesy of Diana West)

17

affected to a variable degree. Multiple studies have attempted to examine the effect of reduction mammaplasty on breastfeeding, and have found widely varying results, with successful lactation outcomes after reduction mammaplasty ranging from zero to 70%, depending upon the type of surgery performed (Widdice, 1993). This wide variability of results reflects a lack of standardization among the criteria used to evaluate lactation outcomes and the methodology used by the investigators, which is important to consider when critically reviewing these studies.

In general, researchers have attempted to quantify lactation outcomes based on the type of surgical approach used. For example, the free nipple graft technique of breast reduction has been found to have decreased successful lactation outcomes when compared to other types of breast reduction techniques (Marshall et al., 1994). This is expected, given that the free nipple graft involves completely severing all nerves, ducts, and blood supply to the nipple and replacing it as a graft. However, this technique is not used as frequently as pedicled techniques, and recent data have found that although nipple sensation is decreased when compared to inferior pedicle breast reduction, some degree of recovery of nipple and areolar sensation occurs after surgery (Ahmed & Kolhe, 2000). This is interesting because it suggests that the neural-hormonal axis can recover after free nipple grafting, which is contrary to the widely held belief that the free nipple graft technique resulted in complete loss of nipple and areola sensation, which would prohibit lactation. In addition, many cases of partial lactation have been anecdotally observed by lactation consultants, and there have been documented reports of mothers who have produced significant quantities of milk (Gillies & Millard, 1957; Townsend, 1974), so it appears that in some cases, a variable degree of lactation may be possible in these women.

As expected, studies examining lactation outcomes after pedicled reduction mammaplasty have shown better outcomes than with free nipple grafting. An early study by Harris et al. queried women who received the inferior pedicle reduction mammaplasty. It reported a 100% lactation rate (defined as any observable lactation), but only a 35% rate of successful breastfeeding (defined as exclusive breastfeeding), and a 65% rate of early cessation or a decision not to breastfeed at all. Although the results are not specific, they do indicate that women who undergo inferior pedicle reduction mammaplasty have the capacity to lactate, although the degree of lactation is unknown (Harris et al., 1992). Similarly, a study by Hefter et al. found that a modified inferior pedicle technique resulted in a 54% successful (without supplementation) lactation rate (Hefter et al., 2003a). This is comparable to the success rate (two weeks with or without supplementation) of approximately 60% in a study of medical pedicle reduction mammaplasty (Cruz-Krochin, 2004). Interestingly, this success rate was not statistically significantly different from the rate observed in matched controls of women who had not undergone breast surgery.

Superior pedicle reduction mammaplasty has also been found to have fairly consistent lactation outcomes. A recent study by Cherchel et al. found a 44% successful lactation rate, as defined by breastfeeding for at least two weeks, with or without supplementation (Cherchel et al., 2007). These results were verified in a study that examined multiple techniques and found successful lactation rates of 60% after superior pedicle, 55.1% after lateral pedicle, 48% after medial pedicle, and 43.5% after inferior pedicle, as defined by breastfeeding for three weeks without supplementation. (Chiummariello et al., 2007).

In perhaps the most comprehensive study to date, Cruz and Korchin compared successful lactation outcomes from women who underwent superior, inferior, and medial pedicle reduction mammaplasty to each other and to matched controls. This study, which defined success as breastfeeding for two weeks with or without supplementation, found a success rate of roughly 60% in each group, and did not find a statistically significant difference in lactation outcomes between any of the groups or the controls who did not undergo surgery (Cruz & Korchin, 2007).

As discussed previously, studies examining successful lactation outcomes after reduction mammaplasty have found widely varying results, which is likely due to non-standardized criteria used to define lactation success, as well as the use of different methodology to conduct the studies. The ideal study would consist of women who had successfully breastfed prior to reduction mammaplasty (as defined by predetermined criteria), then underwent reduction mammaplasty, and later became pregnant and attempted to breastfeed. These women, with a history of lactation success, could serve as their own controls, and thus would allow investigators to more clearly examine the effect of reduction mammaplasty on lactation success. Existing studies seem to show that some degree of lactation is possible in most women who undergo pedicled breast reduction mammaplasty, although the extent of which is unknown. In recent studies, the volume of tissue removed has not been a statistically significant predictor of lactation capability (Hefter et al., 2003, Cruz-Korchin & Korchin, 2006; Cherchel et al., 2006).

It is especially important that clinicians understand that simply having the biophysical machinery intact is not enough to guarantee lactation success. Women who undergo reduction mammaplasty are often overweight or obese, which is a known risk factor for breastfeeding difficulty due to mechanical problems with latching, may experience a decreased response to prolactin during Lactogenesis II (Cruz, 2007), and may suffer from any underlying hormonal contributors to obesity that also affect lactation, such as polycystic ovary syndrome (Marasco et al., 2000), diabetes (Hartmann & Cregan, 2001), or hypothyroidism (Marasco, 2006). When coupled with any difficulties stemming from reduction mammaplasty, these women may be in need of additional support to successfully breastfeed. Numerous studies have documented the importance of having a supportive care team, including input from the doctors and nurses, as well as lactation personnel, as being essential to successful lactation after breast surgery (Chiummariello et al, 2007; Hefter et al., 2003; Brzozowski et al., 2000; Deutinger & Deutinger, 1990). These studies have also documented that discouragement from medical personnel can be a direct cause of breastfeeding failure. Thus, to maximize lactation outcomes in post reduction mammaplasty patients, a knowledgeable and supportive care team must be in place.

Structural Changes in the Surgically Reduced Breast

Many mothers who have had breast reduction surgery lament the fact that during pregnancy their breasts return to their previous size, or even grow larger. A recent study found that at two years post reduction, pregnancy and breastfeeding resulted in a statistically significant increase in the distance between the inferior border of the areola and the inframammary fold, a condition known as pseudoptosis (Cruz-Korchin, 2006). In addition to pregnancy, weight gain can also cause breast enlargement and lead to a ptotic breast. A small proportion of women who choose to undergo reduction mammaplasty in adolescence may have juvenile gigantomastia, a benign disorder of the breast in which one or both of the breasts undergo a massive increase in size during adolescence. This cohort of women is especially prone to recurrence and may require repeat surgical correction or medical therapy (Baker et al., 2001). An important consideration that may be consoling for any post-reduction surgery mother who experiences breast growth after pregnancy is that if she had not had the surgery, the increased breast growth would have occurred from her original breast size, which would have increased her discomfort.

Common Reduction Mammaplasty Techniques

There are many different surgical approaches to reduction mammaplasty. In general, the indications for each approach depend on the patient's anatomy, the surgeon's preference and experience, and the patient's goals. Even standardized techniques vary greatly from surgeon to surgeon. In general, the different pedicles can be used with the different skin incisions, so it is not possible to identify the complete surgical approach by external examination. The discussion of the surgical approaches that follows in this monograph are highly simplified, and are described based on their relevance to lactation.

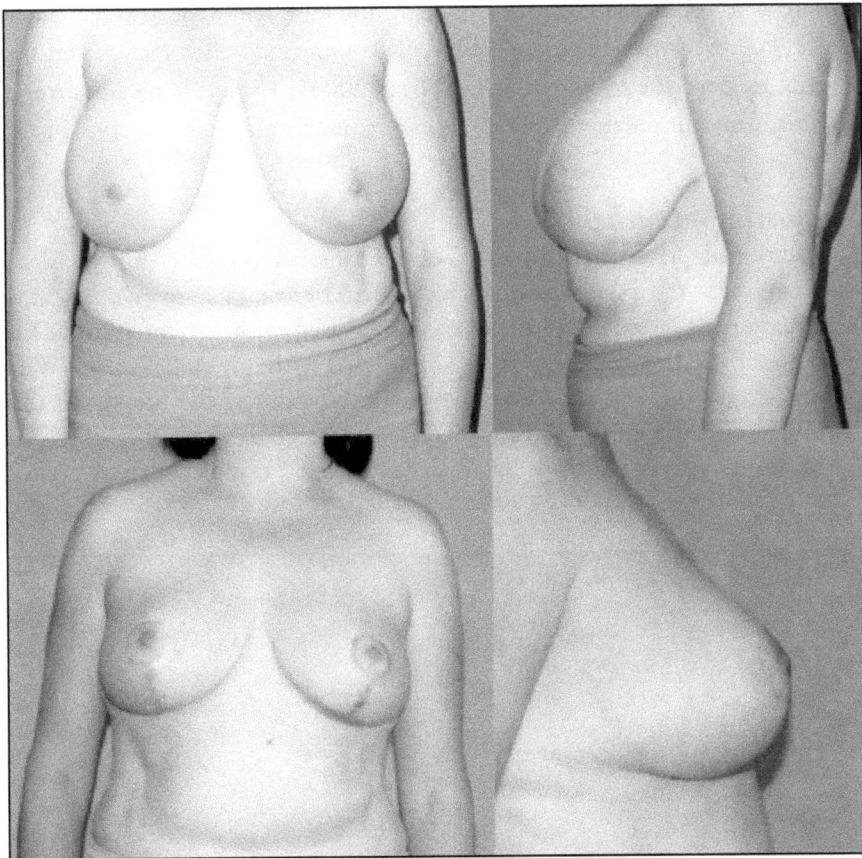

Figure 4. Breast reduction --From cup size F (top left and right) to cup size C (bottom left and right) using the central pedicle technique; significant hypertrophic scarring on the left breast; bottom left and right photos at six months post-op. (Photo courtesy of Diana West)

Liposuction

One surgical technique favored for a subset of women who require only minimal reduction and who do not have significant ptosis is breast reduction by liposuction alone. This process is attractive in that it causes minimal scarring and nerve damage; however, it is usually suggested that this technique be used only for reductions of two or fewer cup sizes (Spear, 2005). Additionally, it is usually best to avoid this technique in younger women who have a higher parenchyma to fat ratio (Nahai, 2008). Liposuction can also be used as an adjunct to other techniques of breast reduction.

Typically, one or more small incisions are made in the breast, the liposuction cannula is passed repeatedly back and forth, and fat is removed. This technique can be improved with the use of ultrasonic equipment, which may permit the surgeon to avoid the mammary lobes (Spear, 2005). Using a blunt liposuction cannula can minimize trauma to breast parenchyma and preserve future function.

Surgical Approaches

As mentioned previously, there are several different types of skin incisions used to access the breast parenchyma, the most common of which is the Wise pattern/inverted T, which is classically used with the inferior pedicle (McKissock) technique, although it can be used with any pedicle. The Wise pattern is very versatile and can be used reliably with any size breast. In this technique, the breast is marked extensively preoperatively, including the inframammary fold, midclavicular line, and classic "keyhole" pattern. Next,

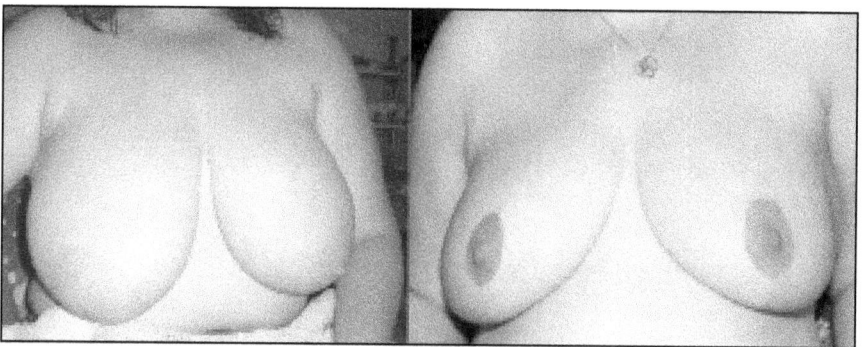

Figure 5.   Breast reduction--Before (left) and after (right); inferior pedicle; right nipple now partially inverted, created difficulty breastfeeding; partial milk supply. (Photo courtesy of Diana West)

the pedicle is deepithelialized and skin flaps are raised. At this point, there are several options for the surgeon to resect the parenchyma, including the "central mound" technique which involves shaping the breast based on a round block of parenchyma. The nipple-areola complex and pedicle are then transposed vertically, and the skin flaps are lowered to support this move. Finally, excess skin is incised from the skin flaps as well as from the new nipple location, and the incisions are closed. This technique results in a scar shaped like an "inverted T" or an anchor.

Another common type of skin incision used in reduction mammaplasty is the vertical scar pattern, frequently used in conjunction with the medial pedicle. This technique is also versatile, although its use is limited to small to moderate reductions (Kryger, 2007). The markings for this technique are different as well, and consist of marking the new nipple location and the borders of the flaps. The remaining steps of the procedure are similar to those for the Wise pattern; however, the shaping and resection of the breast parenchyma is different, and the final scar is in the form of a vertical line.

A third type of skin incision is the circumareolar incision, otherwise known as the Benelli incision. This technique involves making an incision around the perimeter of the areola to access the breast parenchyma (Nahai, 2008). Skin resection is also performed circumareolar, and the incision is typically closed with a purse-string closure which may flatten the areola. Visualization is somewhat limited by virtue of the small incision, and consequently this technique is typically used only for smaller reductions. Variations of this incision use mesh to support and maintain the breast shape. Other variations use a periareolar incision rather than a complete circumareolar incision.

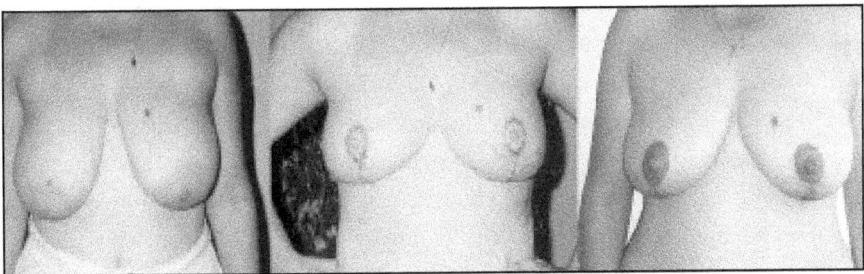

Figure 6. Breast reduction--Before (right), three days post-op (middle), and 13 years later (right); inferior pedicle; mother breastfed two children with 5% milk supply; note pigmentation around vertical incisions. (Photo courtesy of Diana West)

Pedicled reduction mammaplasty

The term "pedicle" refers to the flap of tissue that carries the blood supply to the nipple-areola complex. The most commonly used pedicles are the inferior pedicle (often used with the Wise pattern reduction mammaplasty) and the medial pedicle (frequently used with the vertical scar pattern reduction mammaplasty), although theoretically the pedicle could be created in any direction. Keeping the pedicle intact is a vital component to pedicled reduction mammaplasty. If the pedicle is damaged or made too small, partial or total nipple necrosis may result. This is a devastating complication and may require free nipple grafting to correct, which is likely to be highly detrimental to lactation.

Breast amputation and free nipple graft reduction mammaplasty

Breast amputation with free nipple grafting is rarely performed, and is typically only performed in women with extremely large breasts who would not be amenable to pedicled breast reduction due to the fact that the pedicle could not adequately supply blood to the nipple-areola complex. This technique is an appropriate surgery only for women who do not anticipate future lactation (although some lactation may be possible), as the nipple is completely separated from the ducts, blood supply, and innervation, and survives as a graft. This technique is accomplished by complete removal of the nipple from the breast, followed by large scale resection of breast tissue, and is then completed by grafting the nipple to a well-vascularized tissue bed.

Mastopexy

Mastopexy is surgery to lift and reposition the breasts to reduce ptosis, without reducing volume. This surgical technique reshapes and repositions the breasts, resulting in fuller, rounder, and higher breasts. There are several types of mastopexy techniques, such as the crescentic, circumareolar, and inverted T, which are described based on the pattern of skin excised. The indications for each technique are determined by the degree of breast ptosis. Essentially, this surgery involves removing sections of skin and leaving the breast parenchyma intact. Although the nipple is repositioned during mastopexy, the nipple/areolar complex is not separated from the parenchyma and its innervation should remain intact. Thus, damage to lactation should be minimal.

Mastopexy can also be performed in conjunction with augmentation, which may be carried out in one or two stages. In this case, the risks to successful lactation are the same as the risks of each procedure combined, which have been discussed previously.

Nipple Reduction Surgery

Nipple reduction surgery is performed for women with nipples with long shank lengths on one or both breasts, who desire to have them reduced in length. The surgery is primarily cosmetic and not performed to reduce pain or increase functionality. There are many nipple reduction surgical techniques, ranging from amputation of the top of the nipple to a procedure that removes a cylinder of skin around the neck of the nipple in order to insert the nipple more deeply into the breast. In most cases, lactation is not affected as neither the fourth intercostal nerve nor the ducts within the nipple are severed. The main risk to lactation is from scar tissue that may constrict or obscure the duct openings and hinder milk flow. The surgery may be combined with reduction or augmentation mammoplasties. In such cases, diminishment of lactation functionality is more likely to be related to the mammaplasty than the nipple reduction.

Nipple Enlargement Surgery

Nipple enlargement surgery is performed for a woman who desires to increase the size of her nipples, even though in many cases, they may be normal in projection and shape. There are several techniques to enlarge nipples, usually incorporating tissue grafts. There is a risk of scarring that could potentially obstruct the ducts, and the graft placement could obstruct the ducts as well. However, in most cases, nipple and lactation functionality are unaffected.

Inverted Nipple Release Surgery

Nipple inversion may be congenital or acquired as a result of nipple or ductal trauma or previous breast surgery. Congenital inversion is thought to be due to either exceptionally short ducts or fibrous adhesions that constrict the nipple, drawing it inward. There are several grading systems that are used to classify the degree of inversion, one of which is described below (Han & Hong, 1999):

- **Grade I:** The nipple can be everted easily and maintains projection. The nipples have minimal fibrosis beneath the nipple. Manual manipulation or a simple buried purse-string suture is adequate to achieve protrusion. Lactation is not impacted.
- **Grade II:** The nipple can be everted with moderate difficulty, but does not maintain projection, retracting back into the breast. The majority of inverted nipples fall into this classification. These nipples have moderate

fibrosis beneath the nipple. Surgical treatment involves dissection of the nipple to release fibrotic bands. Lactiferous ducts are preserved and lactation is not impacted.

- **Grade III:** It is difficult or impossible to evert the nipple manually. This is the least frequently encountered grade of nipple inversion. There is severe fibrosis at the base of the nipple so that it is impossible to sever all the fibrotic bands without also severing ducts, particularly in the central portion of the nipple, which can significantly impact lactation. Over time, recanalization of the ducts can regain partial or full functionality, although the degree of recovery is unknown.

Many different surgical techniques to correct inverted nipples have been described in the literature, dating back to the late 1800s (Huang, 2003; Stevens, 2004; el-Sharkawy, 1995). In general, these techniques are either duct-sparing or duct dividing. In duct-sparing techniques, nipple eversion is accomplished by prolonged traction of the nipple or by surgical correction, which typically involves making an incision at the nipple base, then bluntly dissecting through the tissue until the restricting ducts are encountered, and, finally, vertically spreading between the ducts to release the fibrous adhesions. Theoretically, these techniques should not affect lactation, as there should be minimal ductal injury. In certain situations, it may be necessary to selectively divide the ducts in order to achieve complete eversion, which may decrease lactation proportionally to the number of ducts divided. Other techniques involve more extensive division of the ducts, which will further decrease lactation.

LACTATION MANAGEMENT IN THE POST-BREAST OR POST-NIPPLE SURGICAL MOTHER

Latching to a breast that has had surgery to the nipple/areolar complex may be difficult for some babies because the nipple/areolar complex may be less full. A deep, asymmetrical approach will maximize milk transfer and minimize nipple trauma. To facilitate latching, some mothers find that using their index finger to push up into the breast helps evert the nipple (the "nipple nudge").

Engorgement during Lactogenesis II can be a significant hurdle when breastfeeding after breast surgery. Despite the cause or the extent of the engorgement and no matter when it is experienced, it is important to relieve the engorgement in a timely manner to avoid damage to functional alveoli, which can permanently reduce lactation capability.

Most mothers with surviving lactation tissue will experience some degree of engorgement following delivery of their first babies. It is often after delivery of the second baby, though, that engorgement becomes pronounced enough to cause serious discomfort and interfere with breastfeeding. This is because the first lactation experience prompted the recanalization and growth of additional lactation tissue, which is then subject to engorgement.

The extent of recanalization bears a direct correlation between the degree of first and subsequent engorgement episodes. Mothers who lactated longer with the first child will usually experience more engorgement following the next delivery as a result of recanalization than those mothers who lactated for only a short time. Engorgement following the third and subsequent births tends to be at least as pronounced as it was the previous time and may even be more extensive as a result of further recanalization.

Apart from the pain and discomfort of engorgement, many mothers find that the engorgement experience is made more difficult by healthcare professionals who tend to refer to the swelling as an inevitable result of severed ducts, rather than as proof of functional lactation tissue. Mothers are incorrectly warned about a risk of breast infection due to the mistaken belief

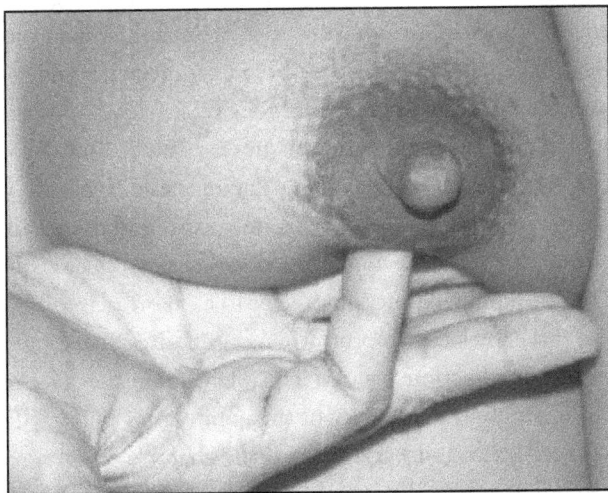

Figure 7. "Nipple Nudge" technique to facilitate latching (Photo courtesy of Diana West)

27

that the engorgement will take longer than normal to resolve since the "milk has nowhere to go" and can become infectious. This is incorrect from the standpoint of both general lactation principles and post-surgical physiology. From the general lactation perspective, engorgement is not a result of a large volume of milk so much as it is swelling of the tissues that surround the glands and ducts in response to a rapid influx of mature milk. Thus, the presence of milk in severed ducts is not responsible for the majority of the engorgement, and so will not have a bearing upon its progress. When the milk is not removed, the alveoli that correspond to the severed ducts atrophy rapidly, so they do not become distended with "backed up" milk and, unless the mother is septic, are not exposed to pathogens and do not progress to infection or abscess.

After Lactogenesis II has resolved, the density of lactation tissue can be assessed by palpation. Adipose tissue is generally less dense than glandular tissue, although fibrocystic tissue can be difficult to differentiate from glandular tissue by palpation. When subglandular implants are present, palpation is most effective and poses the least risk to the implant when done from the top of the breast, with the thumb and fingers on the sides.

If a mother does not experience any fullness at all during Lactogenesis II, this can indicate that her prolactin levels are too low or that the prolactin has not been able to affect milk production, or it may mean that she does not have many viable, intact lobes to produce milk. Occasionally, some mothers experience unequal engorgement between their breasts, again indicating that the viable lactation tissue is present in greater quantities in one breast than the other. Less frequently, some mothers find that they have engorgement only in portions of one or both breasts, but that other areas of the breast remain soft. This is further evidence that little or no viable lactation tissue exists in the non-engorged areas.

The critical component of managing Lactogenesis II in the post-surgical mother is maximizing milk removal to ensure maximum milk production. This may necessitate confirmation that baby is able to remove milk adequately and/or the addition of a pumping regime subsequent to each breastfeeding, particularly during the first three weeks when prolactin receptors are being established.

Initiation of milk ejection is more dependent upon the state of the neural pathways than it is upon the capacity of the mammary gland itself. Of course, even with an excellent milk ejection, the ducts that are not connected cannot express milk and will eventually atrophy. If the nerves of the nipple and areola have been completely severed, particularly the fourth intercostal nerve (assuming reinnervation has not occurred), then milk ejection cannot happen, except as a psychological response or as a result of ingestion or inhalation of synthetic oxytocin. A loss of sensation in the nipple/areolar region indicates the presence of nerve impairment that will negatively impact milk production due to lack of milk removal. Breast compression using external hand pressure to push out any residual milk during breastfeeding or pumping can effectively compensate, minimizing the impact.

The prevalent advice for women who have had breast surgery is to "wait and see what their lactation capability is when their babies are born." This is somewhat of an oversimplification in that it is predicated upon the assumption that milk production can be easily estimated, that it does not fluctuate, and that it cannot be altered. In actuality, milk production is often inaccurately estimated from unreliable criteria; it fluctuates according to hormonal influences and milk removal; and it can be altered by galactagenic medications and increased milk removal.

It is usually in the first few weeks postpartum that mothers determine if there is a requirement for supplementation. Supplementation is not inevitable after breast or nipple surgeries; a significant number of mothers do not need to supplement at all. But for a great many others, it is a necessary component of breastfeeding.

Unless the ducts within the nipple/areola complex were completely severed during the surgery, the chances are good that a mother will be able to produce at least some colostrum. Her baby should have the maximum opportunity to receive as much of this precious substance as possible.

Nursing and additional milk removal via hand expression or pumping with a rental-grade pump as often as possible during the first three weeks will allow her breasts to create as many prolactin receptors as possible, ensuring that her milk supply is maximized to its complete potential.

In order to assess the baby's milk intake, it will be necessary for the parents to be vigilant in tracking their baby's progress. They can do this most efficiently by recording diaper output and monitoring weight. Should clear evidence of insufficient stooling or rapid weight loss be present, immediate supplementation is warranted. Once the baby has had his immediate nutritional needs met, it is important to rule out mechanical breastfeeding problems as the cause of inadequate milk production. Apart from slight tenderness in the first few days, breastfeeding should never hurt. If it does, it means that there is a problem with the way the baby is positioned, latched, or how he suckles the breast. Many mothers find they have poor milk production early on because of positioning, latching, or suckling problems related to alterations in breast structure resulting from their surgeries. The challenge for the lactation consultant will be devising creative strategies to compensate for the inadequacies.

The timing of supplementation depends upon the baby's degree of weight loss. The greater the degree of weight loss, the more critical it is to begin immediate supplementation. Conversely, the less the weight loss, the more room there is to determine if, when, and how much supplementation may be necessary.

Some post-surgical mothers find that their babies gain adequately, and they are able to entirely avoid supplementation in the first few days. After that time, though, their babies' rate of growth slows, and they are forced to reevaluate the necessity of supplementation. A need for late supplementation may be caused by the transition from the endocrine-stimulated lactation system to the autocrine-stimulated lactation system over the first few weeks. A mother can initially have adequate milk production because her milk is being created more from the hormones her body is generating than from the demand that is placed upon it. When the body slowly stops creating hormones automatically, the lactation system becomes more and more dependent upon milk removal and nerve stimulation. At this point, milk production can decrease if the milk removal and stimulation is not adequate to sustain it. The inadequate stimulation is usually not because the mother is not breastfeeding enough, but rather because the nerves in her nipple/areola complex were damaged during her surgery and cannot relay the proper stimulation messages to the lactation system.

The objective in supplementation is augmenting nutritional intake as conservatively as possible to permit the mammary system to produce milk to its fullest capacity, while still assuring that the baby is provided sufficient nutrition and hydration to gain well. It is important to be sensitive to the likelihood that learning supplementation is necessary will be disappointing to mothers who had been hopeful that they would have a full milk supply.

Many mothers who have had breast or nipple surgery increase their inherent milk production capabilities by strategies that involve increased milk removal and/or taking galactagogues (herbal and prescription medications that increase milk production). Increased milk removal is accomplished by methods such as frequent feedings, pumping with a hospital-grade electric pump after feedings, and breast compressions while pumping and nursing. There are many herbal galactagogues that seem to be effective in increasing milk production to varying degrees. Goat's rue, shatavari, fennel, fenugreek, nettle, and alfalfa are reputed to be effective for many post-surgical mothers, particularly when taken in tincture form, which is generally more potent than dried herbs taken in capsule form. Adequate milk removal is essential when galactagogues are employed in order to avoid milk stasis.

Prescription galactagogues, such as domperidone (Motilium®) and metoclopramide (Reglan®), have the ability to increase prolactin and usually result in a more dramatic increase in milk production than herbs. Metoclopramide has a long history of effectiveness in increasing milk production with adequate dosages (up to 15 mg TID) (Hale, 2006; Budd et al., 1993; Ehrenkranz & Ackerman, 1986; Gupta & Gupta, 1985; De Gezelle et al., 1983; Kauppila et al., 1981). However, it crosses the blood-brain barrier and can affect the central nervous system, causing symptoms of depression or dyskinesia (Gabay, 2002). Postpartum women are at particular risk for these side effects (Rodgers, 1992). For this reason, it is not recommended that metoclopramide be taken for longer than three weeks (Hale, 2008).

Domperidone, in contrast, has been demonstrated by many research studies and many hundreds of thousands of lactating women worldwide to be both safe and effective in increasing milk production (Gabay, 2002; da Salva et al., 2001; Brown et al., 2000; Cheales-Siebenaler, 1999; Petraglia et al., 1985; Maddern, 1983; Cann et al., 1983; Hofmeyr & van Iddeking, 1983). The usual dose to increase milk production is 80-120 mg/day taken 20mg QID or 30mg TID/QID. Unlike metoclopramide, it does not cross the blood-brain barrier and, therefore, is unlikely to cause central nervous system symptoms (Gabay, 2002). A recent 2007 study by Reddymasu of 120 mg daily for gastrointestinal dysfunction demonstrated excellent safety. Diabetic patients with digestion problems have used up to 120 mg daily for as long as 12 years without significant side effects (Prakash & Wagstaff, 1998; Soykan et al., 1997). However, research is needed to study the ramifications of long-term use in breastfeeding mothers and babies.

Increases in milk production from the use of galactagogues usually occur within four to seven days, although some women see an increase as soon as two days. Because prolactin levels are already high in the very early postpartum period, galactagogues that increase prolactin are likely to be ineffective before Lactogenesis II (Hansen et al., 2005). When discontinuing prescription galactagogues, it is important to reduce the dosage in gradual increments by no more than 25 percent every 14 days.

SUPPLEMENTATION TO MAXIMIZE BREASTFEEDING

The objective in supplementation is augmenting as conservatively as possible to permit the mammary system to produce milk to its fullest capacity, while still assuring that the baby is provided sufficient nutrition and hydration to gain well. It is important for the lactation consultant to be sensitive to the likelihood that learning supplementation is necessary will be disappointing to mothers who had been hopeful that they would have a full milk supply.

Supplementation Methods

Supplementation options are comprised of combinations of variables of two factors: lactation capability and feeding method. A mother's lactation capability will fall somewhere on a continuum of a full milk supply, a partial milk supply, or no milk supply at all. Feeding method options encompass feeding at the breast, feeding at the breast with an at-breast supplementer, and feeding with artificial feeding devices. The method chosen to feed the baby will depend upon the mother's milk production, the feeding method most appealing to her in terms of comfort and convenience, and her baby's preferences.

At-Breast Supplementation

Mothers who have had breast surgery and who have an incomplete milk supply may choose to supplement at the breast in order to maintain maximum sucking stimulation and enhance milk production. Feeding the baby at the breast with an at-breast supplementer conveys the greatest benefit to the baby, as well as the mother, and allows them to enjoy the harmonious quality of breastfeeding. This type of supplementer employs a plastic bag or bottle that hangs around the neck by a cord. Extending from the bag or bottle is a tube that is placed on top of the nipple and possibly taped in place. As the baby nurses from the breast, supplement is delivered through the tube.

Supplementing a baby's complete nutritional requirement at the breast requires more effort in some ways than bottle-feeding, but it is often more rewarding. Of course, if the mother has no milk at all, the baby does not receive the benefits of human milk. However, he does receive the advantage of better oral and facial development as a result of the suckling motions unique to breastfeeding, as well as better hand-eye coordination as a result of switching from side to side during feedings. Most importantly, though, the baby who is supplemented completely at the breast is able to enjoy all the benefits of the intimate, deeply satisfying emotional bond that comes naturally to the breastfeeding couple. And even though little or no milk is present, these babies are usually willing to nurse without the supplementer for comfort.

Using an at-breast supplementer can be overwhelming to some mothers. If the mother is feeding her baby exclusively at the breast, for the most part, she will be the only one who can feed the baby, both day and night, which is comforting for some women and confining for others. The at-breast supplementer also must be cleaned, prepared, and filled before each feeding. Using it is a learned skill for both mother and baby, and not all mothers and babies find that it works well for them. An at-breast supplementer is contraindicated when baby cannot latch well. It is sometimes more difficult to use an at-breast supplementer at night, although many mothers find they do not need to supplement at night because their milk production is higher then.

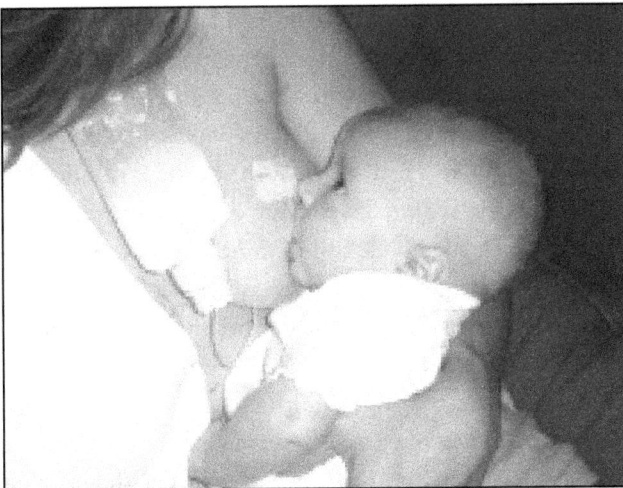

Figure 8. At-breast supplementation (Photo courtesy of Diana West)

Combined Supplementation Methods

Some mothers who have compromised milk production find that they are not comfortable using an at-breast supplementer. They may have tried it and not liked it, or they may never have used it at all. Instead of supplementing at the breast, these mothers nurse their babies at the breast, but also supplement the feeding with a bottle or alternative feeding device, either before or after breastfeeding. Even among those mothers who find at-breast supplementers work well for them, there may be times when using a bottle or alternative feeding device is more convenient than using the at-breast supplementer. Some mothers who use an at-breast supplementer in conjunction with bottles find it more comfortable to feed the baby at the breast when they are at home and feed the baby with a bottle when out in public due to the cumbersome nature of preparing the at-breast supplementer prior to feeding. As long as the baby is adept at using both the human and the artificial nipple, this combined feeding method can work well.

Bottles

Supplementation by bottle is the best choice for some mothers. Bottles are easy to use, convenient, and socially acceptable. While there is a risk of nipple confusion and flow preference that could jeopardize the breastfeeding relationship, there are ways that bottles can be used to support breastfeeding and reduce these risks by using it in a way that is similar to how baby latches to the breast.

Use a Slow-Flow Nipple – To minimizing flow preference, a slow-flow nipple or product that uses an inner chamber to regulate flow should be used. Since the flow from the breast doesn't tend to increase over time, slow-flow nipples continue to be best even when baby gets older.

Hold Baby Upright to Feed – When the bottle is parallel with the floor, the flow from the bottle is slower, reducing flow preference (Kassing, 2002). There is no need to keep the nipple full of milk, nor is swallowing air an issue, because air tends to come right back up naturally as baby burps.

Use a Round Nipple – Ultrasound studies show that round nipples with a broad base encourage babies to latch deeply, extend the tongue, and cup it around the nipple with relaxed lips (Smith et al., 1988). Although flattened-tip orthodontic nipples are often recommended, babies tend to retract their tongues while sucking on them, the opposite of what should happen on the breast (Nowak, 1994). In addition to reducing milk transfer, this type of tongue movement can cause abraded, sore nipples when baby breastfeeds.

Help Baby Latch Deeply to the Bottle – To help baby latch deeply to the bottle, it should be offered pointed up toward the ceiling, with the side of the nipple stroked downward across baby's lips to trigger a wide gape. Then the base of the nipple should be moved to his lower lip and rolled downward into his mouth.

Pace Feedings – Babies feed better when bottle-feedings are periodically paused or paced, simulating the way that breastfeeding babies slow down in between milk ejections. After a few minutes of sucking or if baby's forehead and eyes show signs of stress, he should be tipped forward gently until the milk runs out of the bottle nipple, without removing the nipple from his mouth. This helps baby retain control of the feeding, reminds him to stop when he is full, and helps him to better coordinate sucking, swallowing, and breathing.

Offer Bottle Before Breastfeeding – While traditional wisdom is that bottles should be given only after breastfeeding so that baby sucks actively to remove the most milk, a hungry baby may have less patience for a breast with low supply and may stop trying without taking all the available milk. As a result, they take increasing amounts by bottle and milk production diminishes. Alternatively, babies who quench their initial hunger and thirst with a limited amount of supplement before breastfeeding tend to have more patience feeding at the breast and breastfeed longer even if the flow is slow, removing more milk and increasing milk production. They also learn to associate the euphoria of fullness with the breast rather than the bottle, while the mother has the satisfaction of a contented, "milk drunk" baby falling asleep at her breast. When it happens the other way around, it can undermine her confidence so that she breastfeeds less.

The key to this technique is giving about one-fourth to one-half ounce (7 to 15 ml) less than the amount baby usually needs or takes. If too much is given, baby will not be hungry enough to feed well or long enough at breast. If too little is given, he may not have the patience to nurse. When he looks relaxed or finishes the bottle, whichever comes first, the mother should switch to the breast. If he fusses and seems to want more of the supplement after breastfeeding, she should give it to him, but finish at the breast, even if for just a minute or two. It may take a few days of trial and error to determine the best amount. As more milk is removed and produced, the mother may be able to gradually decrease the amount of the supplement.

Finger-Feeding

When supplementation must be away from the breast, finger-feeding can be used to feed the supplement with a device attached to the finger. This allows parents to avoid giving an artificial nipple, while still allowing baby to suck, which is important physiologically and psychologically. It also allows the baby to have the feeling of human skin during his feeding, which can be comforting. Moreover, it allows him to suck in a similar way to breastfeeding, by keeping his tongue down and forward over his gums, with his mouth wide and jaw forward. Supplementation by finger-feeder is more time consuming than using a cup or other supplementation device and for this reason is best used as a temporary method.

POST-SURGICAL COMPLICATIONS AFFECTING BREASTFEEDING

Scar Tissue

Some breast pain felt by post-surgical mothers, especially during their first lactation experience, can be attributed to scar tissue from surgery. If the scar tissue obstructs the ducts, it can block milk removal. Occasionally, scar tissue can form adhesions to the ducts directly below the nipple, which may pull the nipple towards the breast and cause nipple inversion. When post-surgical mothers have sharp, stabbing breast pain, their physicians may mistakenly attribute the cause of the pain to scar tissue. The mothers may be told there is nothing that can be done about it and the pain is something to be suffered through. In fact, the actual cause of this type of pain is more likely to be either shallow latching or bacterial infection, which are treatable. Therefore, it is important to rule out the more common causes of breast pain in lactating women before attributing it conclusively to scar tissue formation.

Nipple Blanching

It seems to be common for post-surgical mothers to experience a phenomenon that is otherwise rare among breastfeeding mothers, called blanching or nipple vasospasm. Blanching occurs when either the tip of the nipple or the entire nipple becomes rigid, squeezing out all blood and turning completely white. After some time, it may turn blue, and then the nipple will relax and erythema will flush the entire nipple as the blood returns. Some mothers experience only blanching and erythema. Nipple vasospasm is typically very painful, often including numbness, burning, and tingling, possibly with radiating deep breast pain. It can last several minutes and occur frequently, even in between feedings. It is frequently misdiagnosed as a candidal infection.

It is not known why post-surgical mothers experience blanching so commonly. It may be a result of blood supply disruption or nerve trauma to the nipple/areola complex during the surgery. It also may be a result of shallow latching as a consequence of lack of fullness in the nipple/areolar complex, common to those who have had areolar surgery. Blanching can also be caused by many factors, however, that are unrelated to surgical trauma. At one time, it was thought that the phenomenon was a psychosomatic disorder (Gunther, 1970). It is now a well-known medical disorder and is believed to be caused by physical factors, as well as external physical or chemical causes (Coates, 1992).

Some cases of nipple blanching have been identified by numerous clinical studies as a manifestation of Raynaud's syndrome, a disorder that causes blanching in the extremities (Lawlor-Smith et al., 1997). Raynaud's Syndrome usually affects extremities, such as fingers and toes, in persons who are not lactating, but it can also affect coronary, pulmonary, ocular, gastrointestinal, penile, placental, and cerebral blood vessels. In nursing mothers, though, it seems to affect the nipples. Mothers who experience true Raynaud's syndrome have experienced this disorder before breastfeeding as blanching in other parts of the body. They may have primary Raynaud's syndrome with no other symptoms or secondary Raynaud's syndrome, which is caused by an underlying autoimmune or connective tissue disorder.

In mothers who do not have Raynaud's syndrome, blanching may be caused by either external physical or chemical factors. Ankyloglossia, with resulting tight jaw and clamping, can precipitate blanching, as can poor latching and positioning techniques (Genna, 2007). Exposure to cold can also precipitate nipple blanching. Some drugs, such as thophylline, terbutaline, epinephrine, norepinephrine, serotonin, nicotine, and caffeine are known to cause vasoconstriction, which can manifest in the nipple (Lawrence & Lawrence, 1999).

The treatment of nipple blanching depends on the cause of the blanching. When it is caused by Raynaud's syndrome, blanching can be improved by the use of food supplements, such as calcium and magnesium, as well as evening primrose oil (gamma linoleic acid), and fish oil (eicosapentanoic acid and docosahexanoic acid). Unfortunately, it can take up to six weeks to see improvement with these supplements.

When the discomfort from nipple blanching is severe, a prescription medication may be warranted, despite the original cause of the blanching. The most commonly prescribed drug for the treatment of nipple blanching is nifedipine, which is a calcium channel blocker (Page, 2006). It has been shown to be clinically effective in reducing nipple blanching fifty to ninety-one percent of the time. It passes into the milk at a rate of under five percent, which presents virtually no risk to the nursing child. The side effects that are most commonly seen from use of this drug are headache, flushing, dizziness, rapid heartbeat, and edema in the extremities (Hale, 2008; Riordan, 2004).

Nipple blanching caused by poor positioning, latching, or suckling techniques is resolved by improvements to those techniques; nipple blanching caused by ankyloglossia is resolved by a frenotomy (Genna, 2007). Nipple blanching caused by exposure to cold can be prevented by keeping the entire body warm at all times, as it is not enough to keep just the nipples warm. When it has already occurred, however, applying warm compresses to the nipple and/or gently squeezing blood back into the nipple can relax the spasm enough to stop the blanching and pain.

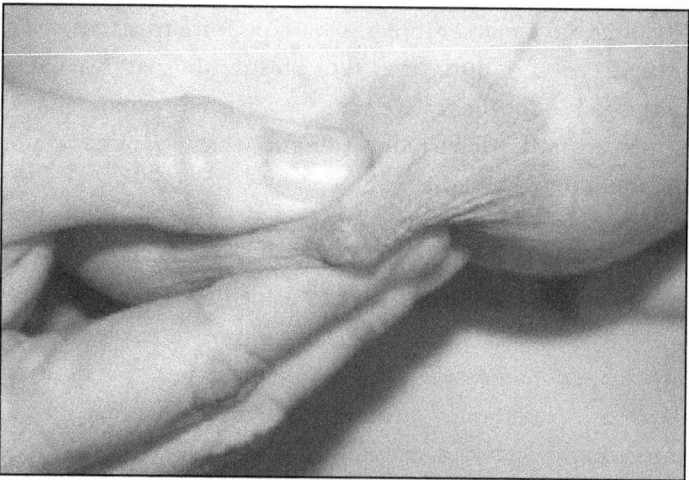

Figure 9. "Vasospasm Squeeze" technique to temporarily resolve vasospasm (Photo courtesy of Diana West)

EFFECTIVE COUNSELING OF MOTHERS WHO HAVE EXPERIENCED BREAST OR NIPPLE SURGERY

Mothers with impaired milk production are in particular need of reassurance by means of an explicit comment from their healthcare professional that asserts awareness of the superiority of breastfeeding and commitment to helping them successfully reach their breastfeeding goals. In discussing breastfeeding with a mother who has had breast or nipple surgery, it is important to be neither overly optimistic about the chance of exclusive breastfeeding nor pessimistic regarding the mother's likelihood of breastfeeding at all. Mothers should be encouraged to celebrate even the smallest milestones. A healthcare professional has a unique opportunity by virtue of the authority of his or her credentials to encourage mothers to understand that while it may not always be possible to breastfeed exclusively after breast or nipple surgery, most mothers can have a satisfying breastfeeding relationship, even with supplementation, and there are many methods of increasing milk production (Kakagia, 2005). It is also important for mothers to understand that it is normal to have mixed feelings about using supplemental feeding devices or breast pumps.

The following recommendations are effective in counseling mothers who wish to breastfeed after breast surgery.

Note Prenatal Breast Changes to Predict Lactation Outcome

In recording a history during a patient consultation, it is important to note the presence or absence of breast changes during pregnancy (enlargement, tenderness, areola darkening), as breast growth and development during pregnancy is correlated with maturation of lactation tissue (Neifert, 1990). Practitioners should ascertain the nipple sensitivity of each breast to assess the likelihood of milk ejection impairment. Also note any other factors that could potentially further decrease milk production (hormonal dysfunction, infertility, persistent copious lochia, etc.).

Facilitate Identification of Breastfeeding Goals

For many mothers who have had breast or nipple surgery, embarking upon the breastfeeding journey is a decision that is made without a great deal of information, primarily because there are few sources for information about breastfeeding after breast or nipple surgery. As she progresses through the stages of lactation, encountering difficulties that she did not know to anticipate, it can be very difficult for her to maintain motivation.

One of the most important services a healthcare professional can provide to a mother who is breastfeeding after breast or nipple surgery is to help her understand and identify her breastfeeding goals by listening to her concerns without judgment. Taking the time to consider alternatives and decide what is important to her may be very enlightening. She may find that she has an unsuspected passion for breastfeeding, or she may find that deep in her heart she does not truly want to breastfeed. You may also be able to help her realize that breastfeeding is not "all or nothing" and that she can adjust the elements of breastfeeding so that it is reasonable for her. Becoming attuned to her own values will give her an outcome to work toward that is perfectly suited to her needs. Having the insight of the mother's values will also help you know how to tailor your lactation consulting perspective to most effectively help her meet her goals.

Facilitate Education about Normal Breastfeeding

It is essential for post-surgical mothers to learn all they can about the normal course of breastfeeding. There are many reliable resources for breastfeeding information; books such as *Breastfeeding Made Simple: Seven Natural Laws for Nursing Mothers* (Mohrbacher & Kendall-Tackett, 2005); international board-certified lactation consultants (IBCLC); mother-to-mother support groups; local classes offered by healthcare providers; and support from experienced breastfeeding mothers among friends and family. Becoming knowledgeable about the "normal" breastfeeding process and issues will help mothers in their experience of breastfeeding after breast and nipple surgeries. They will require a thorough understanding of positioning and latch techniques, including effective ways to position their babies at the breast to facilitate deep latching.

Encourage Mothers to Employ Breastfeeding-Friendly and Breastfeeding Knowledgeable Healthcare Professionals

It is important for mothers to identify and employ breastfeeding friendly and knowledgeable professionals before they need them. The prenatal time is ideal to make calls or ask breastfeeding friends for names of lactation consultants, obstetricians, midwives, and pediatricians. In breastfeeding after breast or nipple surgery, it is important to work with professionals who have a sound knowledge of and experience in lactation. Professionals who believe that formula is "just as good" as human milk and breastfeeding, may not help mothers work through the issues they will face and can actually undermine their efforts with incorrect advice. On the other hand, mothers must be open to the possibility of supplementation and the professionals they consult must be able to determine when this is truly necessary.

Use a Breastfeeding Friendly and Breastfeeding Knowledgeable Healthcare Facility

Finding a breastfeeding-friendly hospital or birthing center is also critically important to breastfeeding success. The length of a mother's stay in the hospital or birthing center should be as short as possible so that she can minimize separations from her baby, as well as unnecessary interventions. Although she may feel that she needs to rest and recuperate from the birth, it is crucial that she keep her baby with her so that she can nurse frequently and on demand, and prevent the use of artificial nipples or pacifiers, which can interfere with the development of her baby's sucking skills. Rooming-in can actually result in better rest for both the mother and the baby by reducing her stress level and encouraging harmonious nursing patterns (Yamauchi & Yamanouchi, 1990). Provided they have been taught the correct means of assessing the baby's intake, being at home will be the most comfortable and restful place for both mother and baby.

Facilitate Affordable Alternatives

Breastfeeding after breast or nipple surgery can be very expensive at a time when new families are already experiencing the harsh realization that the costs of having a new baby can quickly mount. There may be ways that you can help families find affordable alternatives for the breastfeeding aids they require that may very well enable them to continue breastfeeding when they might not have been able to otherwise do so. Even something as simple as writing a letter to help her obtain insurance reimbursement for your services or supplies may make a tremendous difference in the budget of a new family.

Facilitate Appreciation of the Milk Produced

For many mothers who wish to breastfeed after breast or nipple surgery, breastfeeding begins with an expectation that either she will produce a full milk supply or she will bottle-feed. It can be very discouraging when she discovers that she does have milk, but not a full supply. Helping her accept that supplementation is positive because it allows her to continue breastfeeding will be difficult until she understands that every drop of her milk and every moment spent at the breast are of unequaled value to her baby. Developing a profound appreciation for the superiority of her milk and breastfeeding in any amount is essential for her ability to maintain a sufficient level of motivation to persevere in breastfeeding. Educating the mother about ways to maximize her milk production will also empower her to gain some control over her unique breastfeeding situation, thereby decreasing her level of anxiety and fear.

Discuss Birthing Methods that Minimize Interventions

Many studies have shown that medications, including epidurals, especially epidurals containing bupivacaine, during childbirth can significantly inhibit the sucking abilities of newborns by causing the baby to be sleepy and somewhat uncoordinated for a significant period after birth (Kroeger et al., 2004). This very period after birth, however, is a critical window of time to begin breastfeeding which cannot begin until baby is alert and able to latch on properly. This is not to say that there are never circumstances that warrant the use of drugs during birth, but rather that whenever possible, avoiding or minimizing their use will maximize the baby's initial sucking abilities, which are so important for establishing the milk supply. If an epidural is used during labor, it certainly will not make breastfeeding impossible, but will only mean that it may be necessary to pay closer attention to any latching problems that are experienced and to seek help to remedy them.

Preparing for the birth by attending classes in birthing methods that focus on avoiding the use of medications during labor can enhance a mother's chances of having a drug-free birth.

Share Resources about Breastfeeding after Breast and Nipple Surgery

Mothers who are breastfeeding after breast or nipple surgery often are not aware of the many resources for information and support available to them. The healthcare professional is in an excellent position to share resources that will facilitate the experience of breastfeeding after breast surgery. Help the mother explore the many options that are available to make breastfeeding possible. These resources may include a recommendation to read relevant books, such as *Defining Your Own Success: Breastfeeding After Breast Reduction Surgery* (West, 2001) or *The Breastfeeding Mother's Guide to Making More Milk* (West & Marasco, 2008); sharing website addresses, such as the Breastfeeding After Breast Reduction website (www.bfar.org), Low Milk Supply website (www.lowmilksupply.org), and Mothers Overcoming Breastfeeding Issues website (www.mobimotherhood.org); or referral to a knowledgeable healthcare professional, such as an international board certified lactation consultant (IBCLC), a directory of which can be found at www.ilca.org.

Mothers should also be encouraged to attend mother-to-mother support meetings, even if they are supplementing with bottles. The support and encouragement at such meetings can be instrumental in maintaining motivation and identification as a breastfeeding mother.

SUMMARY

Any breast or nipple surgery can significantly impair lactation functionality, depending upon the location, number, and orientation of the incisions, the degree of destruction of parenchyma, and the extent of damage to nerves critical to lactation. Functionality is also affected by the integrity of the parenchyma prior to surgery, the post-operative course, the time interval between the surgery and the lactation event, other lactation experiences between the surgery and this lactation event, breastfeeding management, as well as the mother's attitude toward breastfeeding. It is likely that milk production can be increased by many psychological, mechanical, and chemical devices. When milk production cannot be increased to the point of full lactation, many mothers find that they can still have very satisfying breastfeeding relationships by supplementing in ways that maximize milk production and the time the baby spends at the breast.

REFERENCES

Ahmed A, Kolhe, P. Comparison of nipple and areolar sensation after breast reduction by free nipple graft and inferior pedicle techniques. Br J Plast Surg. 2000 Mar;53(2):126-9.

Aillet S, Watier, E, Chevrier, S, Pailheret, J, Grall, J. Breast feeding after reduction mammaplasty performed during adolescence. Eur J Obstet Gynecol Reprod Biol. 2002 Feb 10;101(1):79-82.

American Academy of Pediatrics. Policy Statement. Breastfeeding and the Use of Human Milk. Pediatrics. 2005 Feb;115(2):496-506.

American Society for Aesthetic Plastic Surgery. 2007 Statistics. Cosmetic Surgery National Data Bank.

Baker S, Burkey B, Thornton P, LaRossa D. Juvenile gigantomastia: presentation of four cases and review of the literature. Ann Plast Surg. 2001 May;46(5):517-25.

Banbury J, Yetman R, Lucas A, Papay F, Graves K, Zins J. Prospective analysis of the outcome of subpectoral breast augmentation: sensory changes, muscle function, and body image. Plast Reconstr Surg. 2004 Feb;113:701-7:discussion 708-11.

Bedard P, Keon W, Brais M, Goldstein W. Submammary skin incision as a cosmetic approach to median sternotomy. Ann Thorac Surg. 1986 Mar;41(3):339-41.

Berlin C. Silicone breast implants and breast-feeding. Pediatrics. 1994;94(4):547-9.

Buescher E. Anti-inflammatory characteristics of human milk: how, why, where. Adv Exp Med Biol. 2001;501:207-22.

Brody G. Lactation after augmentation mammaplasty. Obstet Gynecol. 1996; 87(6):1062-3.

Brown T, Fernandes P, Grant L, Hutsul J, McCoshen J. Effect of parity on pituitary prolactin response to metoclopramide and domperidone: implications for the enhancement of lactation. J Soc Gynecol Investig. 2000 Jan-Feb;7(1):65-69.

Brutel de la Riviere A, Brom G, Brom A. Horizontal submammary skin incision for median sternotomy. Ann Thorac Surg. 1981 Jul;32(1):101-4.

Brzozowski D, Niessen M, Evans H, Hurst L. Breast-feeding after inferior pedicle reduction mammaplasty. Plast Reconstr Surg. 2000 Feb;105(2):530-4.

Budd S, Erdman S, Long D, Trombley S, Udall J. Improved lactation with metoclopramide: a case report. Clin Pediatr. 1993;32(1):53-7.

Cann P, Read N, Holdsworth C. Galactorrhoea as side effect of domperidone. Br Med J. (Clin Res Ed) Apr 30 1983;286(6375):1395-6.

Caputy G, Flowers R. Copious lactation following augmentation mammaplasty: an uncommon but not rare condition. Aesthetic Plast Surg. 1994 Fall;18(4):393-7.

Cheales-Siebenaler N. Induced lactation in an adoptive mother. J Hum Lact. 1999;15(1):41-3.

Cherchel A, Azzam C, De May A. Breastfeeding after vertical reduction mammaplasty using a superior pedicle. J Plast Reconst & Aesth Surg. 2007;60:465-70.

Chiummariello S, Cigna E, Buccheri E, Dessy L, Alfano C, Scuderi N. Breastfeeding after reduction mammaplasty using different techniques. Aesth Plast Surg. 2008 Mar-Apr;32(2):294-7.

Coates M. Nipple pain related to vasospasm in the nipple? J Hum Lact. 1992;8(3):153.

Collins E, Kerrigan C, Kim M, et al. The effectiveness of surgical and nonsurgical interventions in relieving the symptoms of macromastia. Plast Reconstr Surg. 2002 Apr 15;109(5):1556-66.

Cruz N, Korchin L. Lactational performance after breast reduction with different pedicles. Plast Reconstr Surg. 2007;120(1):35-40.

Cruz-Korchin N, Korchin L. Effect of pregnancy and breast-feeding on vertical mammaplasty. Plast Reconstr Surg. 2006;117(1):25-9.

Cruz-Korchin N, Korchin L. Breastfeeding after vertical mammaplasty with medial pedicle. Plast Reconstr Surg. 2004;114(4):890-4.

Da Silva O, Knoppert D, Angelini M, Forret P. Effect of domperidone on milk production in mothers of premature newborns: a randomized, double-blind, placebo-controlled trial. CMAJ. 2001;164(1):17-21.

David F. Lactation following primary radiation therapy for carcinoma of the breast. Int J Radiat Oncol Biol Phys. 1985 Jul;11(7):1425.

De Gezelle H, Ooghe W, Thiery M, Dhout M. Metoclopramide and breast milk. Eur J Obstet Gynecol Reprod Biol. Apr 1983;15(1):31-6.

Deutinger M, Deutinger J. Breast feeding following breast reduction-plasty and mastopexy? Geburtshilfe Frauenheilk. 1990 Mar;50(3):220-2.

Deutinger, M, Dominag E. Breast development and areola sensitivity after submammary skin incision for median sternotomy. Ann Thorac Surg. 1992 Jun;53(6):1023-4.

Deutinger M, Deutinger J. Breast feeding after aesthetic mammary operations and cardiac operations through horizontal submammary skin incision. Surg Gynecol Obstet. 1993 Mar;176(3):267-70.

Didie E, Sarwer D. Factors that influence the decision to undergo cosmetic breast augmentation surgery. J Womens Health (Larchmt). 2003 Apr;12(3):241-53.

Ehrenkranz R, Ackerman B. Metoclopramide effect on faltering milk production by mothers of premature infants. Pediatrics. 1986;78(4):614-20.

el Sharkawy A. A method for correction of congenitally inverted nipple with preservation of the ducts. Plast Reconstr Surg. 1995 May;95(6):1111-4.

Escobar P, Baynes D, Crowe J. Ductosopy-Assisted Microdochectomy. Int J Fertil. 2004;49(5):222-4.

FitzJohn T, Williams D, Laker M, Owen J. Intravenous urography during lactation. Br J Radiol. 1982;55(656):603-5.

Frey M. A new technique of reduction mammaplasty: dermis suspension and elimination of medial scars. Br J Plast Surg. 1999 Jan;52(1):45-51.

Gabay M. Galactogogues: medications that induce lactation. J Hum Lact 2002 Aug;18(3):274-9.

Genna C. Supporting sucking skills in breastfeeding infants. Sudbury, MA:Jones and Bartlett Publishers, 2007.

Gilles H, Millard D. The principles and art of plastic surgery. Boston: Little Brown, 1957:412.

Gunther M. Infant feeding. London: Methuen, 1970.

Gupta A, Gupta P. Metoclopramide as a lactogogue. Clin Pediatr. 1985;24(5):269-72.

Hale T. Anesthetic medications in breastfeeding mothers. J Hum Lact. 1999;15(3):185-94.

Hale T. Medications and mothers' milk. 13th edition. Amarillo, TX: Hale Publishing, 2008.

Han S, Hong Y. The inverted nipple: its grading and surgical correction. Plast Reconstr Surg. 1999 Aug;104(2):389-95; discussion 396-7.

Hansen W, McAndrew S, Harris K, Zimmerman M. Metoclopramide effect on breastfeeding the preterm infant: a randomized trial. Obstet Gynecol. 2005 Feb;105(2):383-9.

Harris L, Morris S, Freiberg A. Is breast feeding possible after reduction Mammaplasty? Plast Reconstr Surg. 1992 May;89(5):836-9.

Hartmann P, Cregan M. Lactogenesis and the effects of insulin-dependent diabetes mellitus and prematurity. J Nutri. 2001;131(11):3016S-20S.

Hefter W, Lindholm P, Elvenes O. Lactation and breast-feeding ability following lateral pedicle mammaplasty. Br J Plast Surg. 2003 Dec;56:746-51.

Helewa M, Levesque P, Provencher D, Lea R, Rosolowich.V, Shapiro H. Breast cancer, pregnancy, and breastfeeding. J Obstet Gynaecol Can. 2002 Feb;24(2):164-80.

Henriksen T. Incidence and severity of short-term complications after breast augmentation: results from a nationwide breast implant registry. Ann Plast Sur. 2003 Dec;51(6):531-9.

Higgins S, Haffty B. Pregnancy and lactation after breast-conserving therapy for early stage breast cancer. Cancer. 1994 Apr 15;73(8):2175-80.

Hofmeyr G, van Iddeking B. Domperidone and lactation. Lancet. 1983;1(8325):647.

Huang W. A new method for correction of inverted nipple with three periductal dermofibrous flaps. Aesthetic Plast Surg. 2003 Jul-Aug;27(4):301-4.

Hurst N. Lactation after augmentation Mammaplasty. Obstet Gynecol. 1996 Jan; 87(1):30-4.

Illingworth P. Diminution in energy expenditure during lactation. Br Med J. (Clin Res Ed) 1986 Feb 15;292(6518):437-41.

Kakagia D, Tripsiannis G, Tsoutsos D. Breastfeeding after reduction mammaplasty: a comparison of 3 techniques. Ann Plast Surg. 2005 Oct;55(4):343-5.

Kauppila A, Kivinen S, Ylikorkala O. Metoclopramide increases prolactin release and milk secretion in puerperium without stimulating the secretion of thyrotropin and thyroid hormones. J Clin Endocrinol Metab. 1981 Mar;52(3):436-9.

Kroeger M, Smith L. Impact of birthing practices on breastfeeding: Protecting the mother and baby continuum. Sudbury, MA:Jones and Bartlett Publishers, 2004.

Kryger Z, Sisco M. Practical plastic surgery. Austin, TX: Landes Bioscience, 2007.

Kubik-Huch R, Gottstein-Aalame N, Frenzel T, et al. Gadopentetate dimeglumine excretion into human breast milk during lactation. Radiology. 2000 Aug;216(2):555-8.

Lawlor-Smith L, Lawlor-Smith C. Vasospasm of the nipple – a manifestation of Raynaud's Phenomenon. Br Med J. 1997;314:644-5.

Lawrence R, Lawrence R. Breastfeeding: A guide for the medical professional. 5th edition. St. Louis, Missouri:Mosby, 1999.

Love S. Dr. Susan Love's breast book. 3rd ed. Cambridge, MA:Perseus Publishing, 2000.

Maddern G. Galactorrhea due to domperidone. Med J Aust. 1983;2:539-40.

Marasco L. The impact of thyroid dysfunction on lactation. Breastf Ab. 2006;25(2):9, 11-12.

Marasco L, Marmet C, Shell E. Polycystic Ovary Syndrome: A connection to insufficient milk supply? J Hum Lact. 2000;16(2):143-8.

Marshall D, Callan P, Nicholson W. Breastfeeding after reduction mammaplasty. Br J Plast Surg. 1994 Apr;47(3):167-9.

Michalopoulos K. The effects of breast augmentation surgery on future ability to lactate. Breast J. 2007;13(1):62-7.

Modfid M, Klatsky S, Singh N, Nahabedian M. Nipple-aerola complex sensitivity after primary breast augmentation. Plast Reconstr Surg. 2006;117:1694.

Mohrbacher N. The breastfeeding answer book. 3rd Rev Ed. Schaumburg, Illinois:La Leche League International, 2004.

Mohrbacher N, Kendall-Tackett K. Breastfeeding made simple: Seven natural laws for nursing mothers. Oakland, CA:New Harbinger; 2005.

Nahabedian M, McGibbon B, Manson P. Medial pedicle reduction mammaplasty for severe mammary hypertrophy. Plast Reconstr Surg. 2000 Mar;105(3):896-904.

Nahai F, Nahai F. MOC-PSSM CME Article: Breast Reduction. Plast Reconstr Surg. 2008;121(1S) MOC-PS:1-13

Nakamura K, Irie H, Inoue M, Mitani H, Sunami H, Sano S. Factors affecting hypertrophic scar development in median sternotomy incisions for congenital cardiac surgery. J Am Coll Surg. 1997 Sep;185(3):218-23.

Neifert M, Seacat J, Jobe W. Lactation failure due to insufficient glandular development of the breast. Pediatr. 1985 Nov;76(5):823-8.

Neifert M. Breastfeeding after breast surgical procedure or breast cancer. NAACOGS Clin Issu Perinat Womens Health Nurs. 1992;3(4):673-82.

Neifert M, DeMarzo S, Seacat J, Young D, Leff M, Orleans M. The influence of breast surgery, breast appearance, and pregnancy-induced breast changes on lactation sufficiency as measured by infant weight gain. Birth. 1990 Mar;17(1):31-8.

Nielsen S, Matheson I, Rasmussen J, Skinnemoe K, Andrew E, Hafsahl G. Excretion of iohexol and metrizoate in human breastmilk. Acta Radiol. 1987;28(5):523-6.

Nommsen-Rivers L. Cosmetic breast surgery - is breastfeeding at risk? J Hum Lact. 2003;19(1):7-8.

Nowak A, Smith W, Erenberg A. Imaging evaluation of artificial nipples during bottle feeding. Arch Pediatr Adolesc Med. 1994 Jan;148:40-2.

Page S, McKenna D. Vasospasm of the nipple presenting as painful lactation. Obstet Gynecol. 2006 Sept;108(3 pt 2):806-8.

Petraglia F, De Leo V, Sardelli S, et al. Domperidone in defective and insufficient lactation. Eur J Obstet Gynecol Reprod Biol. May 1985;19(5):281-7.

Pezzi C, Kukora J, Audet I, Herbert S, Horvick D, Richter M. Breast conservation surgery using nipple-areolar resection for central breast cancers. Arch Surg. 2004 Jan;139(1):32-7.

Prakash A, Wagstaff A. Domperidone. A review of its use in diabetic gastropathy. Drugs. 1998 Sep; 56(3):429-45.

Reddymasu S, Soykan I, McCallum R. Domperidone: review of pharmacology and clinical applications in gastroenterology. Am J Gastroenterol. 2007;102(9):2036-45.

Riordan J. Breastfeeding and human lactation. 3rd ed. Sudbury, MA: Jones and Bartlett Publishers, 2004.

Rodgers C. Extrapyramidal side effects of antiemetics presenting as psychiatric illness. Gen Hosp Psychiatry. 1992 May;14(3):192-5.

Rofsky N, Weinreb J, Litt A. Quantitative analysis of gadopentetate dimeglumine excreted in breast milk. J Magn Reson Imaging. 1993 Jan-Feb;3(1):131-2.

Scott-Conner C. Diagnosing and managing breast disease during pregnancy and lactation. Medscape Womens Health. 1997 May;2(5):1.

Schlenz I, Kuzbari R, Gruber H, Holle J. The sensitivity of the nipple-aerola complex: An anatomic study. Plast Reconstr Surg. 2000;105:905.

Semple J, Lugowski S, Baines C, Smith D, McHugh A. Breast milk contamination and silicone implants: preliminary results using silicon as a proxy measurement for silicone. Plast Reconstr Surg. 1998;102:528-33.

Shaw W, Orringer J, Ko C, Ratto L, Mersmann C. The spontaneous return of sensibility in breasts reconstructed with autologous tissue. *Plast Reconstr Surg.* 1997;99: 394-9.

Smith W, Erenbert A, Nowak A. Imaging evaluation of the human nipple during breast-feeding. Am J Dis Child. 1988;142:76-8.

Soykan I, Sarosiek I, McCallum R. The effect of chronic oral domperidone therapy on gastrointestinal symptoms, gastric emptying, and quality of life in patients with gastroparesis. Am J Gastroenterol. 1997 Jun;92(6):976-80.

Spear S (ed). Surgeries of the breast: principles and art. Philadelphia, PA: Lippincott-Raven, 2006.

Spear S, Low M, Ducic I. Revision augmentation mastopexy: indications, operations, and outcomes. Ann Plast Surg. 2003 Dec;51(6):540-6.

Spigset O. Anaesthetic agents and excretion in breast milk. Acta Anaesthesiol Scand. 1994 Feb;38(2):94-103.

Stevens W, Fellows D, Vath S, Stoker D. An integrated approach to the repair of inverted nipples. Aesthetis Surg Journal. 2004;24(3)211-5.

Strom S, Baldwin B, Sigurdson A, Schusterman M. Cosmetic saline breast implants: a survey of satisfaction, breast-feeding experience, cancer screening, and health. Plast Reconstr Surg. 1997 Nov;100(6):1553-7.

Tralins A. Lactation after conservative breast surgery combined with radiation therapy. Am J Clin Oncol. 1995 Feb;18(1):40-3.

Townsend P. Nipple sensation following breast reduction and free nipple transportation. Br J Plast Surg. 1974;27:308.

West D. Defining your own success: breastfeeding after breast reduction surgery. Schaumburg, IL:La Leche League International; 2001.

West D, Marasco L. The breastfeeding mother's guide to making more milk. New York, NY:McGraw-Hill, 2008.

Widdice L. The effects of breast reduction and breast augmentation surgery on lactation: an annotated bibliography. J Hum Lact. 1993 Sep;9(3):161-7.

Yamauchi Y, Yamanouchi I. The relationship between rooming-in/not rooming-in and breast-feeding variables. Acta Paediatr Scand. Nov 1990;79:1017-22.

GLOSSARY

Ablative surgery................ Surgery to excise tissue.

Adipose tissue .... Tissue comprised of fat cells (fatty tissue).

Alveoli .... (individually called alveolus)
The basic unit component of the mammary system, containing specialized cells that produce milk derived from elements of the adjacent bloodstream.

Anastamose .... To join together.

At-breast supplementer..... A supplementation device that supplies supplemental nutrition at the breast while a child is suckling.

Augmentation
    mammaplasty................ Breast enlargement surgery.

Autocrine milk removal.. (also known as supply-and-demand milk production)
The system of milk production that produces milk in direct response to the amount of milk that is removed. It is self-perpetuating, not hormonally-driven.

Axilla .... The arm pit.

Breast compressions.......... Compression of the breast with the thumb on the top of the breast and the fingers beneath while nursing or pumping to move milk through the ducts and simulate milk ejection.

Cannula .... A suction tube used in liposuction surgeries.

Capsular contracture........ A capsule of scar tissue that has formed around a breast implant and is squeezing the implant, distorting the appearance of the breast.

Capsulectomy .... Excision of a capsule of scar tissue that has formed around a breast implant.

Capsulotomy..................... Surgical scoring or cutting of the capsule of scar tissue in order to release its pressure upon the breast implant.

Colostrum	The first clear, yellowish milk produced by the breasts after birth.
Cooper's ligaments	Suspensory connective tissue within the breast.
Diagnostic surgery	Surgery to determine the nature of the physiological dysfunction.
Ducts	Conduits that convey milk through the breast from the milk-producing portions of the gland.
Ductules	Smaller branches of the ductal network.
Endocrine milk production	The initial postpartum lactation process that relies upon hormonal stimulation rather than milk removal for milk production.
Engorgement	The normal postpartum process whereby the mature milk appears suddenly and copiously in the first few days after birth, resulting in tremendous swelling in the breasts. Engorgement can also occur at any time during lactation when a larger amount of milk is produced than removed.
Fasciculi	Bundles of individual nerve fibers surrounded by a perineureum.
Foremilk	The milk the baby receives when he begins suckling. Thin and usually bluish, it is the milk that has accumulated since the last nursing and has a higher protein, but lower fat content than hindmilk.
Galactocele	A milk-filled cyst.
Galactagogue	A substance that increases the milk supply.
Galactagenic	The ability of a substance to increase the milk supply.
Galactorrhea	Spontaneous milk production.
Gigantomastia	Extreme growth of breast tissue.
Hindmilk	The milk actively produced during the feeding after most of the foremilk has been removed. Hindmilk is much higher in fat, which results in a thick, white appearance.
Hypoplasia	A smaller amount of tissue growth than normal.
Hypertrophy	Excessive tissue growth.

Innervation	The nerve supply of a structure.
Intercostal spaces	The regions between the ribs.
Inframammary fold	The junction of the breast and the chest wall.
Intertrigo	Irritant dermatitis caused by tissue edges rubbing.
Lactogenesis II	Transition from the colostrum stage of lactation to mature milk.
Lactogenesis III	Weaning.
Lobuli	Clusters of alveoli.
Mammaplasty	Surgery of the breast (see also reduction Mammaplasty and augmentation Mammaplasty).
Mastectomy	Surgical removal of the breasts and lactation tissue.
Mastopexy	Breast lift without removal of breast tissue.
Mature milk	Milk that has fully transitioned from colostrum.
Milk ejection reflex (MER)	The process by which milk is forcibly expelled from the milk-producing glands, through the ducts, and from the breast.
Myoepithelial cells	Minute muscles that squeeze milk from the alveoli cells.
Neural pathways	The interlacing network of nerve fibers that allows a nerve impulse to follow a myriad number of pathways.
Nipple/areolar complex	The combined anatomical structures of the nipple and areola.
Oncology	The medical specialization of cancer diagnosis and treatment.
Oxytocin	A hormone produced by the pituitary gland that stimulates uterine and lactiferous smooth muscle contractions.
Parenchyma	The functional elements of a structure.
Periareolar	Around the circumference of the areola.
Percutaneous	Through the skin.
Pituitary gland	The endocrine gland that produces prolactin and oxytocin.
Prolactin	A hormone produced by the pituitary gland that influences and promotes lactation.
Ptosis	Sagging.

Reduction mammaplasty ..   Breast reduction surgery.

Reinnervation ....   The process by which nerve segments are regrown.

Sebaceous glands ....   Glands that produce fatty substances known as sebum.

Stroma ....   Tissue that provides a formative structure to the breast.

Transition milk ....   The yellowish breastmilk that is in the process of transitioning from colostrum into mature milk.

Vascularization ....   The establishment of the network of blood veins and arteries.

INDEX

AUTHOR BIOGRAPHIES

Diana West is an international board-certified lactation consultant (IBCLC) in private practice, co-author with Lisa Marasco of *The Breastfeeding Mother's Guide to Making More Milk* (McGraw-Hill, 2008), author of the *Clinician's Breastfeeding Triage Tool* (International Lactation Consultant Association, 2007) and *Defining Your Own Success: Breastfeeding After Breast Reduction Surgery* (La Leche League International, 2001), as well as numerous magazine articles. She has a bachelor's degree in psychology, is a retired La Leche League Leader, a website developer, and administrator of the popular *BFAR.org, LowMilkSupply.org, LactSpeak.com,* and *LactAsk.com* websites. She is Director of Professional Development for the International Lactation Consultant's Association Board of Directors. She and her family raise German shepherd guide dog puppies for the Seeing Eye. Most importantly, Diana mothers her three charming, breastfed sons in partnership with her husband Brad in their home in New Jersey.

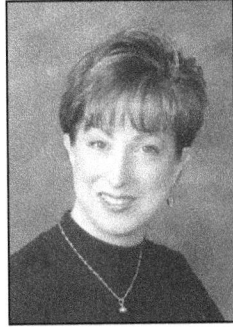

Elliot M. Hirsch, MD, received his BA in Behavioral Biology at Johns Hopkins University, where he graduated with Phi Beta Kappa and Omicron Delta Kappa Honors and received the Curt P. Richter award for outstanding research in Behavioral Biology. Dr. Hirsch attended medical school at the Keck School of Medicine of the University of Southern California, where he won the annual MedSTARS research competition. He graduated with Highest Distinction and was inducted into the Alpha Omega Alpha Honor Society. Dr. Hirsch has authored and co-authored over fifteen peer reviewed journal publications and has given both regional and national presentations. He is currently an integrated Plastic and Reconstructive Surgery resident at Northwestern Memorial Hospital in Chicago, Illinois, where he lives with his wife Jessica and their dog Max.

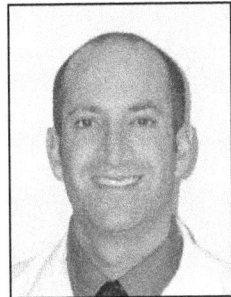